THE COMPLETE PLANT-BASED LOW FODMAP DIET COOKBOOK

A SUPER EASY GUIDE TO BOOST DIGESTIVE HEALTH, MANAGE IBS, IMPROVE GUT HEALTH AND LOSE WEIGHT

CATHERINE JONES

Copyright Page

© 2023 Catherine Jones

Table of Contents

INTRODUCTION

A dietary strategy called the "Plant-Based Low FODMAP Diet" is intended to reduce symptoms of upset stomach, especially in those who have irritable bowel syndrome (IBS) or other gastrointestinal disorders. Fermentable Oligosaccharides, Disaccharides, Monosaccharides, and Polyols, or FODMAPs, are a class of carbohydrates that, in certain cases, can cause symptoms related to the digestive system, including gas, bloating, stomach pain, and abnormal bowel movements.

This diet emphasizes the consumption of plant-derived foods while restricting certain types of carbohydrates that are high in FODMAPs. It combines the ideas of a low-FODMAPS diet with a plant-based diet. Reducing gastrointestinal symptoms without sacrificing vital nutrients is the goal.

Studying FODMAPs and their origins is necessary to comprehend this diet. Foods high in fructooligosaccharides (FODMAPS), including several fruits, vegetables, grains, legumes, and sweets, can make sensitive people's digestive problems worse. As a result, the diet calls for substituting low-FODMAPS items with high-FODMAPS ones, either completely or in moderation.

A plant-based strategy adheres to the low FODMAP criteria and emphasizes a wide range of fruits, vegetables, grains, nuts, seeds, and plant-based proteins. It promotes eating more nutrient-dense plant meals that are less prone to cause upset stomachs.

Careful preparation and familiarity with appropriate food substitutes are necessary for this diet. To ascertain each person's tolerance threshold, there is an elimination phase in which foods high in fructooligosaccharides are temporarily restricted, and a reintroduction phase that follows. Maintaining a low FODMAP diet in conjunction with a plant-based diet guarantees that people get enough nutrition while easing their digestive discomfort.

In the end, comprehending the Plant-Based Low FODMAP Diet entails learning the low FODMAP approach's tenets and putting them to use inside a plant-based dietary framework to relieve digestive discomfort and advance general health. When starting this diet, it is best to speak with a medical practitioner or registered dietitian for individualized advice and assistance.

Benefits of a Plant-Based Approach

Eating a plant-based diet has several advantages for health that go beyond physical well-being. Here are a few main benefits:

Nutrient-Dense Foods: A diet based mostly on plants will usually contain a wide range of vital nutrients, such as vitamins, minerals, antioxidants, and fiber, as well as a variety of fruits, vegetables, whole grains, legumes, nuts, and seeds. These nutrients help prevent disease and support immune system performance and general health.

Decreased Risk of Chronic Illnesses: Research indicates that eating a plant-based diet may reduce your chance of acquiring long-term conditions like obesity, heart disease, high blood pressure, type 2 diabetes, and some malignancies. They are often higher in heart-healthy elements and lower in cholesterol and saturated fats.

Better Digestive Health: Plant-based diets frequently have a high fiber content, which helps maintain a healthy gut microbiota, encourage regular bowel movements, and help with weight management.

Weight management: When well-balanced, plant-based diets naturally have fewer calories and saturated fats than diets heavy in animal products. They can lower the risk of obesity-related disorders by helping with weight management and loss.

Environmental Sustainability: Diets heavy in plant-based foods have less of an impact on the environment than diets heavy in animal products. Because they consume less energy, water, and land, they help to preserve the environment and cut down on greenhouse gas emissions.

Ethical & Animal Welfare: By consuming fewer animal products, a plant-based diet is in line with ethical concerns for animal welfare. Many people choose to follow plant-based diets out of moral obligation to refrain from using animals for food production.

Enhanced Vitality and Longevity: According to certain studies, following a plant-based diet is linked to longer lifespans and a decreased chance of passing away too soon. Plant-based diets are rich in antioxidants and minerals, which support general health and vigor.

Versatility and Culinary Ingenuity: Plant-based diets provide a wide range of dietary options and creative cooking opportunities. By encouraging the exploration of many flavors, textures, and cuisines without mainly relying on materials produced from animals, they foster creativity in the kitchen.

Getting Started: Essential Tools and Ingredients

Having the appropriate supplies and foods on hand can make the transition to a Plant-Based Low FODMAP Diet easier and increase the likelihood that the dietary restrictions will be followed. Below is a summary of the necessary supplies and equipment to get you going:

TOOLS:

Food Scale: Very helpful for measuring exact amounts of components, particularly when reintroducing foods to the diet.

Measuring cups and spoons: Crucial for precise ingredient measurement and portion management.

Food containers are perfect for meal preparation and convenient storage of prepared meals or supplies.

A blender or food processor works well for making fresh ingredient purees, sauces, dips, and smoothies.

Vegetable Spiralizer: Great for using carrots, zucchini, and other low-FODMAPS vegetables to make noodles or ribbons.

Non-stick Cookware: It facilitates cooking with less oil and keeps food from sticking, which makes meal preparation simpler.

Low-FODMAPS Diet Reference Material: Books, websites, or applications that offer thorough lists of foods low-FODMAPS as well as appropriate replacements for certain ingredients.

INGREDIENTS:

Vegetables Low in FODMAPs: Bell peppers, spinach, kale, carrots, cucumbers, tomatoes, and lettuce are a few examples.

Fruits with low fructose monosaccharides: Strawberries, blueberries, oranges, kiwis, bananas, and grapes are good options (in moderation).

Gluten-Free Grains: Low FODMAP grains that are frequently used in diets include quinoa, brown and white rice, gluten-free oats, and corn.

Proteins: Plant-based protein sources include tofu, tempeh, firm tofu, and (in moderation) canned legumes such lentils or chickpeas.

Nuts and Seeds: Low FODMAP choices that contribute nutrition and texture include almonds, sunflower, pumpkin, and chia seeds.

Non-Dairy Milk Substitutes: Lactose-free, rice, or almond milk can be used in place of dairy milk.

Herbs and Spices: You may add flavor without worrying about FODMAPs by using fresh herbs like ginger, paprika, turmeric, and cumin, as well as spices like thyme, parsley, and basil.

Low-FODMAPS Oils: You can cook with olive oil, coconut oil, and other vegetable-based oils.

SECTION 1: BREAKFASTS

Breakfasts are an essential way to start the day full of nutrition and energy. This diet emphasizes the use of plant-based components and low-FODMAPS meals together. Smoothies high in nutrients and easy on the stomach, such as those made with almond milk, spinach, blueberries, and strawberries, provide a reviving start to the day. Breakfast bowls made with quinoa, pumpkin seeds, and raspberries offer a delicious combination of flavors, textures, and vital nutrients that won't upset your stomach.

If you're looking for something savory, a tofu scramble with bell peppers, cumin, and turmeric is a great substitute for regular egg-based meals. Made with lactose-free yogurt or bananas, gluten-free pancakes offer a satisfying breakfast choice that goes well with fresh fruit or a drizzle of maple syrup. Chia seed pudding, made with low-FODMAPS almond milk and garnished with low-FODMAP almonds or raspberries, also makes a filling, high-fiber breakfast that keeps you full all morning.

These breakfast options follow the guidelines of the Plant-Based Low FODMAP Diet while accommodating a range of dietary requirements and tastes. Low FODMAP components are given priority, guaranteeing a satisfying and pleasurable start to the day without sacrificing digestive comfort. Adding these breakfast options to your diet lays the groundwork for maintaining energy levels and fulfilling your nutritional needs in accordance with this specialty diet.

Energizing Morning Smoothies

A Plant-Based Low FODMAP Diet must include Energizing Morning Smoothies, which provide a satisfying and practical breakfast choice. Leafy greens like spinach or kale, low-FODMAPS fruits like strawberries, blueberries, and bananas (in moderation), and a non-dairy base like almond or rice milk are often combined in these smoothies. Occasionally, adding almond butter or chia seeds to a smoothie improves its nutritious value. These colorful mixtures offer a welcome hit of fiber, vitamins, and antioxidants that promote digestive health without causing discomfort. Their adaptability enables inventive mixing, guaranteeing a high-nutrient and simple-to-digest breakfast that suits a variety of palates and dietary requirements.

Low FODMAP Breakfast Bowls

A mainstay of the Plant-Based Low FODMAP Diet, Low FODMAP Breakfast Bowls provide a delicious fusion of tastes, textures, and health benefits. These bowls usually have cooked rice or quinoa as the foundation, with a variety of low-FODMAPS fruits such as raspberries, kiwi, or a small amount of banana on top. Other garnishes could be seeds, such sunflower or pumpkin seeds, which add crunch and a serving of good fats. A dash of cinnamon or a drizzle of maple syrup frequently elevates the flavor profile by adding a hint of sweetness or warmth. With a combination of vital nutrients, these customised bowls offer a filling, easy-to-digest breakfast choice that meets individual tastes and low-FODMAPS recommendations.

Hearty Quinoa Porridge

A satisfying and wholesome breakfast choice that fits inside the parameters of the Plant-Based Low FODMAP Diet is Hearty Quinoa Porridge. This recipe calls for cooked quinoa, a flexible and low FODMAP grain, which is made with almond milk that is lactose-free or another suitable nondairy substitute. Usually, it has a modest amount of maple syrup or a hint of sweetness from a low-FODMAPS fruit, such strawberries, to provide it a well-balanced flavor. This porridge, topped with almonds or pumpkin seeds, has a pleasing texture and a good amount of protein and healthy fats. Packed with fiber, vitamins, and minerals, this warm, adaptable breakfast bowl is a satisfying, low-digestible choice that meets nutritional requirements as well as the desire for a healthy start to the day.

Vegan Pancakes with Berry Compote

A delicious and decadent breakfast option that is in line with the Plant-Based Low FODMAP Diet is Vegan Pancakes with Berry Compote. Typically, mashed low-FODMAPS fruits, including bananas, chia seeds or flaxseed meal, and a gluten-free flour blend are used to make these pancakes. When cooked to a light texture and flavor on a nonstick surface, they are incredibly fluffy.

A delicious berry compote, consisting of low-FODMAPS berries such as blueberries or strawberries that have been gently simmered down with a hint of maple syrup, goes perfectly with these pancakes. This compote naturally sweetens the pancakes and gives them a fruity flavor boost without making your stomach feel queasy.

This breakfast choice fits the nutritional requirements of a Plant-Based Low FODMAP Diet and is high in fiber, antioxidants, and other nutrients. It also makes a delicious morning snack. It addresses dietary requirements as well as taste preferences, providing a tasty and easy way to start the day.

Nutty Chia Seed Pudding

A satisfying and adaptable breakfast choice, Nutty Chia Seed Pudding follows the guidelines of the Plant-Based Low FODMAP Diet. Usually, to make this pudding, you combine chia seeds with a foundation of lactose-free almond milk and refrigerate the mixture until it thickens over night.

Finely chopped low-FODMAPS nuts, like walnuts or almonds, give the pudding a pleasing crunch and a delicious nutty flavor. Some versions could include a dash of cinnamon for extra flavor or a dab of vanilla essence.

This breakfast alternative is a satisfying and nutrient-dense morning meal since it provides an abundance of omega-3 fatty acids, fiber, and protein from the chia seeds and nuts. Convenience is provided by its make-ahead nature and adjustable toppings, like coconut flakes or a handful of raspberries, which provide flavor and texture without interfering with the comfort of the digestive system. All things considered, this chia seed pudding fits both dietary requirements and the need for a healthy start to the day. It is a tasty and gut-friendly complement to a plant-based low FODMAP diet.

SECTION 2: LUNCHES

Plant-based nutrition and comfort for the digestive system are given priority in Plant-Based Low FODMAP Diet lunches. These dishes feature a lot of veggies, tofu, tempeh, and gluten-free grains like rice or quinoa, as well as other low-FODMAPS ingredients. The emphasis is still on creating recipes that are savory and gratifying, but avoiding items high in fructooligosaccharides (FODMAPS) that could cause upset stomachs. Colorful salads, filling stir-fries, inventively stuffed veggies, and rolls or wraps stuffed with colorful, digestive-friendly items are common lunch alternatives. These sandwiches offer a harmony of flavors, textures, and minerals, making it a satisfying and easily digestible midday meal that complies with the Plant-Based Low FODMAP Diet's dietary recommendations.

Rainbow Salad with Lemon-Tahini Dressing

The colorful and nourishing Rainbow Salad with Lemon-Tahini Dressing perfectly captures the spirit of the Plant-Based Low FODMAP Diet. This vibrant salad offers a range of flavors and nutrients with its assortment of low-FODMAPS vegetables, including bell peppers, spinach, cucumbers, and any other desired vegetable arranged in a rainbow-like pattern.

This salad's tangy and creamy Lemon-Tahini Dressing is its pièce de résistance. Made with tahini, a paste made from sesame seeds, and enhanced with fresh lemon juice, oil scented with garlic, and a touch of maple syrup, this dressing has a delicious combination of acidity and creaminess without making you feel queasy.

This salad is full of vitamins, minerals, and fiber from the variety of veggies, in addition to being aesthetically pleasing. The Lemon-Tahini Dressing adds flavor and healthful fats to the dish, making it taste better overall. Following the Plant-Based Low FODMAP Diet, it provides a nutrient-dense, refreshing lunch alternative that is easy on the stomach thanks to its adherence to low FODMAP ingredients.

Tofu and Veggie Stir-Fry

A tasty and filling dish that perfectly captures the spirit of the Plant-Based Low FODMAP Diet is the Tofu and Veggie Stir-Fry. This stir-fry is made using tofu, a flexible plant-based source of protein, along with a variety of low-FODMAPS vegetables such as carrots, bell peppers, bok choy, or any other veggies of your choice. These ingredients provide depth and taste without sacrificing ease of digestion when they are sautéed together in a wok or skillet with aromatic spices like ginger and garlic-infused oil.

A small amount of soy sauce or tamari is usually added to the dish to give it a savory and umami taste in the stir-fry. Utilizing these low-FODMAPS components guarantees a meal that is pleasant to the digestive system and offers a variety of vital nutrients, including as vitamins, minerals, and plant-based proteins.

This stir-fry delivers a vibrant medley of flavors and textures without causing stomach distress, embodying taste and nutrition. It is evidence of the adaptability of plant-based components in the Plant-Based Low FODMAP Diet, providing a filling and healthy dinner choice that puts digestive health and general wellbeing first.

Mediterranean Stuffed Peppers

A tasty and nutritionally balanced dish that adheres to the Plant-Based Low FODMAP Diet is Mediterranean Stuffed Peppers. Usually roasted, these peppers are stuffed with a healthy mixture of low-FODMAPS foods including spinach, quinoa, and Mediterranean herbs.

Herbaceous spices like thyme and oregano provide subtle flavor to the stuffing, giving it a Mediterranean-style flavor. Occasionally, feta cheese or a dollop of lactose-free yogurt are added to boost taste depth and richness without sacrificing digestive comfort.

This recipe offers a filling and aesthetically pleasing supper with a well-balanced combination of flavors and textures. Mediterranean Stuffed Peppers follow the nutritional guidelines of the Plant-Based Low FODMAP Diet and include vital nutrients, such as fiber, vitamins, and minerals, with an emphasis on gut-friendly foods.

Tempeh Tacos with Lime Slaw

With the Plant-Based Low FODMAP Diet, Tempeh Tacos with Lime Slaw offer a colorful and flavorful entrée. The plant-based protein source tempeh, which is seasoned with chili powder and cumin to give the tacos a delicious and aromatic filling, is the star of these tacos.

To go with the tempeh is a spicy lime slaw made with low-FODMAPS veggies like carrots and cabbage and a zesty lime vinaigrette. The tacos' flavor profile is improved by the crisp, citrusy zing from this slaw, all without causing upset stomachs.

The richness of the seasoned tempeh is balanced with the crispiness of the lime-infused slaw in these tacos, which deliver a harmony of flavors and textures. They are a delicious and gut-friendly dinner choice that fits into the Plant-Based Low FODMAP Diet, demonstrating the adaptability of plant-based components while following low FODMAP rules.

Rice Paper Rolls with Peanut Dipping Sauce

The Plant-Based Low FODMAP Diet is supported by the tasty and refreshing Rice Paper Rolls with Peanut Dipping Sauce. These rolls have a light and colorful texture and are made from low-FODMAPS veggies including cucumbers, lettuce, and carrots that have been carefully wrapped in rice paper.

These rolls come with a delicious peanut dipping sauce that is made with tamari, peanut butter, and a touch of ginger. The rolls benefit from the depth and richness of this sauce, which also imparts a blast of savory flavors without sacrificing digestive ease.

The rolls are a delightful treat to consume, a harmonic fusion of crisp, fresh vegetables wrapped in soft rice paper. These rolls, when paired with the tasty peanut dipping sauce, present a pleasant blend of flavors and textures that complies with the Plant-Based Low FODMAP Diet's dietary recommendations while highlighting the variety and acceptability of gut-friendly ingredients.

SECTION 3: DINNERS

The Plant-Based Low FODMAP Diet emphasizes low FODMAP components and serves up tasty, easily digested meals for dinner. These dinners feature a variety of low-FODMAPS vegetables together with gluten-free grains like quinoa or rice, along with a range of plant-based proteins like tofu, tempeh, and legumes. Herbs and spices are frequently used to season food to add flavor without affecting stomach comfort. Crafting foods that are both fulfilling and enjoyable while maintaining a balance of taste, nutrients, and gut-friendly ingredients is still the major focus. These dinner alternatives offer a range of culinary styles and follow the Plant-Based Low FODMAP Diet's nutritional recommendations, so you can have a tasty and comfortable evening meal.

Zucchini Noodles with Avocado Pesto

Within the framework of the Plant-Based Low FODMAP Diet, Zucchini Noodles with Avocado Pesto is a light and nutrient-dense dish. These noodles are a low-FODMAPS substitute for regular wheat-based noodles. They are often made by spiralizing zucchinis into spaghetti-like strands. The creamy avocado pesto, a delicious combination of ripe avocados, fresh basil, a sprinkling of lemon juice, and a dash of garlic-infused oil, is the star of this dish.

The crisp and reviving texture of the barely cooked or raw zucchini noodles nicely pairs with the creamy avocado pesto. Avocados are a great source of healthy fats in this dish, which also provides a good dosage of important nutrients and a filling meal that won't upset your stomach. It's a clever and flexible alternative that emphasizes how flexible plant-based foods can be, and it presents a tasty but gentle dinner option that fits the Plant-Based Low FODMAP Diet's nutritional guidelines.

Lentil Bolognese over Spaghetti Squash

This filling and substantial dish of lentil bolognese over spaghetti squash is ideal for the Plant-Based Low FODMAP Diet. In this dish, spaghetti squash—a low-FODMAPS substitute with a gentle, noodle-like texture—replaces traditional pasta. The lentil Bolognese sauce, the dish's main attraction, is made from cooked lentils simmered with chopped tomatoes, herbs like basil and oregano, and just a touch of garlic-infused oil for flavor depth.

The flavorful lentil Bolognese sauce paired with spaghetti squash makes for a hearty, satisfying supper that won't upset your stomach. This recipe highlights the adaptability of vegetables as a base for traditional recipes and is full of plant-based proteins from the lentils. This meal's mildly flavored profile is in perfect harmony with the tenets of the Plant-Based Low FODMAP Diet, providing a satisfying and nutritious dinner choice that prioritizes taste, nutrition, and ease of digestion.

Roasted Vegetable Curry

Roasted Vegetable Curry is a delicious and nutrient-dense dinner option for the Plant-Based Low FODMAP Diet. It features a variety of low-FODMAPS, perfectly roasted vegetables, like bell peppers, carrots, and zucchini, mixed with a mild and aromatic curry sauce made from coconut milk and infused with fragrant spices like turmeric, cumin, and ginger. The curry offers a delicate balance of creaminess from the coconut milk and a touch of heat from the spices, creating a tasty and comforting dish. It provides a range of necessary nutrients from the assortment of roasted vegetables and the richness of coconut milk while maintaining a gentle profile suitable for digestive comfort. This curry showcases the diversity and flavors of plan

Stuffed Portobello Mushrooms

This meal, stuffed portobello mushrooms, is flavorful and filling and fits into the Plant-Based Low FODMAP Diet. These mushrooms provide as a tasty foundation and are packed with quinoa, spinach, and other low-FODMAPS nutrients. Aromatic spices like thyme or rosemary are frequently used to season this stuffing, giving it a savory and herbaceous flavor profile.

The dish presents a contrast of flavors and textures, with the stuffing's herb-infused taste complemented by the earthy flavor of the mushrooms. Because portobello mushrooms are low in FODMAPs, they can be used in a variety of ways to provide a satisfying and healthy dinner. This recipe offers a combination of vital elements, such as protein from quinoa and vitamins from spinach, while also being easy on the stomach and following the Plant-Based Low FODMAP Diet's nutritional recommendations.This meal, stuffed portobello mushrooms, is flavorful and filling and fits into the Plant-Based Low FODMAP Diet. These mushrooms provide as a tasty foundation and are packed with quinoa, spinach, and other low-FODMAPS nutrients. Aromatic spices like thyme or rosemary are frequently used to season this stuffing, giving it a savory and herbaceous flavor profile.

The dish presents a contrast of flavors and textures, with the stuffing's herb-infused taste complemented by the earthy flavor of the mushrooms. Because portobello mushrooms are low in FODMAPs, they can be used in a variety of ways to provide a satisfying and healthy dinner. This recipe offers a combination of vital elements, such as protein from quinoa and vitamins from spinach, while also being easy on the stomach and following the Plant-Based Low FODMAP Diet's nutritional recommendations.

One-Pot Quinoa Paella

A tasty and practical dish that perfectly captures the spirit of the Plant-Based Low FODMAP Diet is One-Pot Quinoa Paella. This meal uses quinoa, a low FODMAP grain, as the foundation, simplifying the traditional Spanish paella. This dish has a lot of color and taste and is made with a variety of low FODMAP vegetables like tomatoes, peas, and bell peppers.

The quinoa has a rich flavor reminiscent of traditional paella thanks to the infusion of fragrant spices like paprika, saffron, and a tiny bit of oil infused with garlic. This nutritious one-pot meal offers a variety of vitamins and minerals from the veggies as well as protein from the quinoa.

This recipe is an appealing and healthy dinner option because of how easy and convenient it is to prepare in one pot. It demonstrates how versatile plant-based components are in the Plant-Based Low FODMAP Diet, guaranteeing a fulfilling dinner that is both tasty and easy on the digestive system.

SECTION 4: SNACKS AND SIDES

The Plant-Based Low FODMAP Diet includes a variety of tasty and nutrient-dense snacks and sides that can be eaten in between bigger meals or as a way to add flavor to meals. Fresh fruit, almonds (in moderation), rice cakes, and small amounts of specific cheeses (like cheddar or brie) are just a few of the low-FODMAPS foods that make up these snacks and sides. All of these options are in keeping with the recommendations of the diet.

These choices emphasize gut-friendly components that aid in digestion while offering a harmony of tastes, textures, and minerals. Snacks and sides are an important part of a well-rounded Plant-Based Low FODMAP Diet since they help sustain energy levels and provide vital nutrients throughout the day.

Roasted Red Pepper Hummus with Veggie Sticks

Roasted Red Pepper Hummus paired with Veggie Sticks is a tasty and nourishing side dish or snack that is ideal for the Plant-Based Low FODMAP Diet. Usually made with chickpeas, roasted red peppers, tahini, a little lemon juice, and a tiny bit of garlic-infused oil, this savory hummus is mixed to creamy perfection.

When paired with vibrant and crispy vegetable sticks like bell peppers, cucumbers, and carrots, this snack offers a delicious contrast of flavors and textures. The crisp, fresh veggies provide a counterpoint to the rich, savory flavor character of the hummus.

In addition to satisfying appetites, this snack provides a wealth of nutrients, such as fiber, protein, and other vitamins and minerals from the veggies and chickpeas. It is a delicious and gut-friendly alternative that can be eaten as a side dish or as a snack, and it perfectly fits the guidelines of the Plant-Based Low FODMAP Diet.

Spiced Roasted Chickpeas

A delicious snack or side dish that goes well with the Plant-Based Low FODMAP Diet are Spiced Roasted Chickpeas. These delectable chickpeas are seasoned with a mixture of spices, such as cumin, paprika, or cayenne for a little heat, and then they are roasted till crispy perfection.

Roasted chickpeas, which are rich in fiber and plant-based protein, provide a delightful crunch and taste boost without interfering with easy digestion. They are a quick, nutrient-dense snack that keeps you feeling full in between meals.

This snack satisfies taste preferences and provides critical nutrients while adhering to the principles of the Plant-Based Low FODMAP Diet. It is crispy and flavorful. With their taste and nutritious value, these spiced roasted chickpeas are a great addition to any snacking repertoire.

Baked Sweet Potato Fries with Herbed Yogurt Dip

A tasty and filling snack or side dish that fits great with the Plant-Based Low FODMAP Diet is Baked Sweet Potato Fries with Herbed Yogurt Dip. Sweet potatoes are cut into fries and roasted till crispy, with a small amount of oil and seasoning added. High FODMAP items like onion or garlic are usually excluded from the recipe.

This snack delivers a delicious combination of textures and flavors, especially when paired with a cool herbed yogurt dip made from lactose-free yogurt and flavored with fragrant herbs like parsley or chives. The yogurt dip offers a creamy and herbaceous contrast, and the sweet potato fries offer a natural sweetness and a healthy dose of vitamins.

This snack provides a filling and nutritious alternative that doesn't upset the stomach, while still meeting the requirements of the Plant-Based Low FODMAP Diet. It demonstrates how easily basic items may be transformed into a tasty and stomach-friendly snack or side dish.

Low FODMAP Trail Mix

The Plant-Based Low FODMAP Diet is well-suited to the easy and nutrient-dense snack known as Low FODMAP Trail Mix. This mixture usually consists of low FODMAP nuts (almonds, macadamias, etc.), pumpkin or sunflower seeds, and a small quantity of dried fruits (blueberries, cranberries, etc.) that follow low FODMAP serving recommendations.

The combination provides a good amount of protein, healthy fats, and natural sweetness from the dried fruits. It is a healthy and filling between-meal snack that increases energy.

This trail mix accommodates the Plant-Based Low FODMAP Diet's dietary recommendations while providing a practical and portable snack alternative. It does this by avoiding high FODMAP items such as some nuts or excess dried fruits.

SECTION 5: DESSERTS AND TREATS

The Plant-Based Low FODMAP Diet offers a range of delectable desserts and delights that prioritize gut-friendly foods with a hint of decadence. Low FODMAP fruits, such as strawberries, blueberries, or kiwis, are frequently used in these sweets, along with plant-based or lactose-free creams, to create a pleasant and easily digestible sweetness.

Cakes or muffins devoid of gluten that are baked with rice or almond flour and sweetened with maple syrup or low-FODMAPS sweeteners like glucose syrup or stevia are some options. Chia seed puddings with coconut milk and a dash of vanilla might also be served as desserts for a rich, creamy delight.

The goal of these sweets and treats is to satisfy and add just a hint of sweetness without sacrificing stomach comfort. Offering a variety of tasty options that satisfy a sweet desire while putting an emphasis on gut-friendly ingredients, they are consistent with the tenets of the Plant-Based Low FODMAP Diet.

Vegan Chocolate Avocado Mousse

A delicious and health-conscious dessert that is ideal for the Plant-Based Low FODMAP Diet is vegan chocolate avocado mousse. Ripe avocados serve as the foundation for this rich mousse, which substitutes plant-based components for dairy and has a luxurious texture.

This dessert gives a rich and decadent chocolate flavor without using high FODMAP components. It is blended with unsweetened cocoa powder, a dab of vanilla extract, and a small amount of maple syrup or a low FODMAP sweetener. The inherent creaminess of the avocado creates a velvety texture, while the addition of chocolate brings a delicious depth of flavor.

This dessert is rich in nutrients and tastes great. It contains antioxidants from chocolate and healthy fats from avocados. In keeping with the tenets of the Plant-Based Low FODMAP Diet, it offers a creamy, delightful, and guilt-free dessert that doesn't upset your stomach.

Blueberry Almond Crumble Bars

These delicious and nutrient-dense Blueberry Almond Crumble Bars fit the definition of a plant-based, low-FODMAPS treat. A basis for these bars is usually made of almond flour, gluten-free oats, and a low-FODMAPS sweetener like rice malt syrup or maple syrup.

The filling is made up of a layer of frozen or fresh blueberries that have been boiled down to a jam-like consistency and mildly sweetened, giving it a delicious flavor boost without having high FODMAP elements.

A crumbly mixture consisting of the same basic components is used to top the bars; sliced almonds are frequently added for taste and texture. These bars have a crunchy yet tender texture since they are roasted till golden brown.

This dessert delivers a delicious blend of sweet, fruity, and nutty flavors, showcasing the variety of low FODMAP components. It's a filling dessert that satisfies dietary requirements and fits within the Plant-Based Low FODMAP Diet. It tastes incredibly nutritious.

Citrus Infused Fruit Salad

This Citrus Infused Fruit Salad is a bright and cool dessert or snack that fits well with the Plant-Based Low FODMAP Diet. This salad offers a medley of colors and flavors by combining a variety of low-FODMAPS fruits, such as oranges, strawberries, kiwis, and grapes.

Usually, a citrus-infused dressing consisting of freshly squeezed orange or lemon juice, a small amount of maple syrup or a low-FODMAPS sweetener, and maybe a dash of fresh mint for flavor and scent, is drizzled over the fruit.

This dessert is a light and refreshing way to end a meal or a great snack option because it has a blast of natural sweetness and tanginess from the fruits and zesty dressing. It is in line with the tenets of the Plant-Based Low FODMAP Diet, providing a naturally sweet and easily digested dessert that highlights the health benefits of fruits without causing pain to the digestive system.

SECTION 6: BEVERAGES

A wide range of reviving and gut-friendly beverages that focus low FODMAP components while providing flavor and hydration are included in the Plant-Based Low FODMAP Diet. These drinks typically avoid ingredients that are rich in fructose corn syrup (FODMAPS), like some fruits, artificial additives, and sweeteners like honey.

Herbal teas that are calming for the digestive system and naturally low in FODMAPs, such as chamomile or peppermint, could be an option. Drinks may also include plant-based or lactose-free milks, including rice or almond milk, to avoid dairy products that are high in FODMAPs.

Other options include adding slices of low-FODMAPS fruits, such as cucumber, lemon, or lime, to water to add flavor without adding too much FODMAPs. The Plant-Based Low FODMAP Diet's guiding principles are supported by these drinks, which offer a selection of cooling and easily digested drink options that promote hydration without causing pain in the digestive tract.

Ginger Turmeric Tea

Inside the Plant-Based Low FODMAP Diet, Ginger Turmeric Tea is a soothing and health-promoting beverage. Traditionally, hot water is combined with freshly grated ginger and turmeric, which are well-known for their anti-inflammatory and digestive effects.

Occasionally, a squeeze of lemon or a hint of low-FODMAPS sweetener, like maple syrup, is added to improve the flavor without making digestion more difficult. The ginger and turmeric in the tea add a nice spicy taste and a hint of earthiness, while also providing warmth.

This drink is calming and comforting, so it's a great option that follows the guidelines of the Plant-Based Low FODMAP Diet. This is a tasty, easy-to-digest alternative that may have positive effects on your health.

Cucumber-Mint Infused Water

A cool and hydrating choice for the Plant-Based Low FODMAP Diet is Cucumber-Mint Infused Water. For this drink, cucumber slices and fresh mint sprigs are infused into water, allowing their flavors to gently infuse the water without contributing any high-FODMAPS ingredients.

The end product is a refreshing, cool drink with a subtle flavor that tastes like cucumber and mint combined to give a hint of freshness and herbal essence. This naturally flavored water is a great option for staying hydrated without causing discomfort to your digestive system because it doesn't contain any added sugars or components high in FODMAPs.

This drink is in line with the Plant-Based Low FODMAP Diet's tenets and provides an easy and delightful method to up your water intake. It tastes gentle and pleasant and contains no substances that may cause stomach problems.

Berry Blast Smoothie

A tasty and nutrient-rich beverage that is ideal for the Plant-Based Low FODMAP Diet is the Berry Blast Smoothie. Low FODMAP berries like raspberries, blueberries, or strawberries are usually combined with plant-based or lactose-free milk alternatives like almond or coconut milk in this smoothie.

This naturally sweet smoothie is enhanced with a hint of low-FODMAPS sweeteners, like stevia or maple syrup, without sacrificing digestive comfort.

The combination of berries offers a powerful punch of antioxidants, vitamins, and minerals, and the nondairy milk gives it a creamy texture without being heavy in fructose.

This smoothie is a hydrating and nourishing choice that satisfies cravings for fruit while following the Plant-Based Low FODMAP Diet's dietary restrictions. It's a gratifying and easy-on-the-gut beverage option that prioritizes flavor, nutrients, and ease of digestion.

Iced Green Tea with Citrus

A tasty and nutritious beverage that goes well with the Plant-Based Low FODMAP Diet is iced green tea with citrus. In order to make this beverage, steep the green tea, let it cool, then chill and serve it over ice.

In order to add a hint of tanginess without making digestion more difficult, it frequently contains a citrus twist, like a slice of lime or lemon. This drink retains its integrity and provides hydration and a gentle caffeine boost from the green tea without the use of additives or sweeteners with high fructose monohydrate content.

This iced green tea, with its blend of antioxidants and a hint of zesty citrus, is a hydrating and flavorful beverage that complies with the Plant-Based Low FODMAP Diet's dietary guidelines while also being free of ingredients that may cause upset stomachs.

Breakfast

SECTION 7: PLANT-BASED, LOW-FODMAP DIET RECIPES

BREAKFAST LOW-FODMAP DIET RECIPES

Quinoa Porridge with Cinnamon Apples

Ingredients

1 cup red quinoa, rinsed and drained

2 cups water

1 tablespoon butter

1 apple - peeled, cored and diced

½ teaspoon salt

1 tablespoon ground cinnamon

2 tablespoons maple syrup

⅓cup sliced almonds

1 ½ cups almond milk

1 tablespoon half-and-half cream, or to taste (Optional)

Directions

Step 1

Bring the quinoa and water to a boil in a saucepan over high heat. Reduce heat to medium-low, cover, and simmer until the quinoa is tender and the water has been absorbed, about 15 to 20 minutes.

Step 2

Melt the butter in a large skillet over medium heat. Add the apple, and sprinkle with salt, cinnamon, and maple syrup. Stir in the almonds; cook and stir until the apple is hot and beginning to soften, 2 to 3 minutes. Pour in the almond milk and half-and-half cream; continue cooking until hot. Stir in the hot quinoa, and cook a few minutes before serving.

Pumpkin Quinoa Bread

Ingredients

1 (15 ounce) can pumpkin puree

1 cup light brown sugar

1 cup white sugar

¾ cup canola oil

3 eggs

2 ½ cups whole wheat flour

1 teaspoon ground cinnamon

1 teaspoon ground nutmeg

¾ teaspoon baking soda

¾ teaspoon baking powder

¾ teaspoon salt

½ teaspoon ground allspice

½ teaspoon ground cloves

1 cup cooked quinoa

1 cup chopped walnuts

½ cup dried cranberries

Directions

Step one

Preheat oven to 350 degrees F (175 degrees C). Grease and flour a 9x5-inch loaf pan.

Step two

Whisk pumpkin, brown sugar, white sugar, canola oil, and eggs together in a bowl until smooth. Sift flour, cinnamon, nutmeg, baking soda, baking powder, salt, allspice, and cloves together in a separate bowl. Stir flour mixture, a little at a time, into pumpkin mixture until batter is smooth; fold in quinoa, walnuts, and cranberries. Pour batter into prepared loaf pan.

Step 3

Bake in the preheated oven until top of loaf springs back when lightly touched, 50 to 60 minutes.

Tofu Scramble Wraps

Ingredients

Breakfast Potatoes:

2 cups peeled and chopped sweet potatoes

½ cup chopped onion

½ cup chopped green bell pepper

1 medium lime, juiced

1 tablespoon coconut aminos

¼ teaspoon garlic powder

¼ teaspoon ground black pepper

Tofu Scramble:

1 (14 ounce) package extra-firm tofu, drained

1 tablespoon nutritional yeast

1 tablespoon coconut aminos

½ teaspoon garlic powder

¼ teaspoon ground black pepper

1 pinch black salt

1 tablespoon water, or more if needed

4 ounces seitan, cut into chunks

1 small tomato, chopped

2 small avocados, diced

4 (8 inch) flour tortillas

Directions

Step 1

Preheat the oven to 450 degrees F (230 degrees C). Line a baking tray with parchment paper or a silicone liner (such as Silpat®).

Step 2

Combine sweet potatoes, onion, bell pepper, lime juice, coconut aminos, garlic powder, and pepper for potatoes in a medium bowl, stirring so that everything is evenly coated. Transfer to the prepared baking tray.

Step 3

Cook in the preheated oven until crisp and tender, 30 to 40 minutes, stirring halfway through cooking time.

Step 4

While the potatoes are cooking, crumble the tofu into a large, nonstick pan. Add nutritional yeast, coconut aminos, garlic powder, pepper, and black salt. Cook over low heat, adding 1 tablespoon of water at a time if the tofu starts to stick, for 10 minutes. Add seitan and tomato, and cook until everything is warmed through, about 20 minutes.

Vegan Tofu Scramble Breakfast Sandwiches

Ingredients

2 tablespoons vegetable oil

1 (12 ounce) package firm tofu, drained

¾ cup canned fire-roasted tomatoes, drained

1 medium red bell pepper, diced

½ medium yellow onion, diced

2 cloves garlic, minced

1 ½ tablespoons nutritional yeast

1 ½ tablespoons soy sauce

½ teaspoon red pepper flakes

½ teaspoon paprika

¼ teaspoon ground turmeric

1 pinch salt to taste

1 tablespoon vegan mayonnaise, or to taste

5 sandwich buns, split

1 cup fresh spinach

1 avocado, sliced

Directions

Heat oil in a large pan over medium heat. Crumble tofu into roughly 1-inch pieces and add to the pan. Cook, stirring occasionally, for 5 minutes. Add canned tomatoes and cook until excess liquid has evaporated, 5 to 10 minutes. Add bell pepper and onion and cook until onion is translucent, about 5 minutes. Add garlic, nutritional yeast, soy sauce, red pepper flakes, paprika, turmeric, and salt. Cook and stir for 2 minutes more

Step 2

Spread mayonnaise over sandwich buns and top with tofu mixture, spinach, and avocado.

Whole Oat Groats with Cherries, Plums, Pistachios & Homemade Almond Milk

Ingredients

Homemade almond milk

1 cup almonds

1 1/2 cups water

a little love, sure, why not

Oat Groats with First Of The Season Plums & Cherries, Nuts & Dried Figs

1 cup oat groats, soaked overnight with 1 tablespoon lemon juice

2 in-season plums, if small, one if using larger stoned fruit of your choice, pitted and chopped

10 cherries, pitted

2 tablespoons shelled pistachios

3 tablespoons raw almonds, chopped

6 dried mission figs, chopped

1/2 cup or so homemade almond milk. Recipe above.

 Prepararion

rinse your oats, get 'em into the pot. Cook on low for, oh, I don't know, 20 minutes? Until the grains are al dente. If they are al dente and there is still a lot of liquid left in the pot, don't fret. You would rather have too much liquid in the pot than two little and have to add more during the cooking process, which can lend to uneven cooking and undercooked grains. Simply drain the excess liquid and discard. When I made this yesterday, I had 1/3 more liquid left that I had to drain off.

When your oats are al dente, stir in your sliced up figs, and about 1/3 cup the homemade almond milk (recipe above). More if you like it creamier. Cook for a couple of minutes until the figs begin to dissolve. Stir the dissolving figs into the porridge to sweeten it.

I can't believe this is the last step. Spoon into bowls. top with all of your awaiting goodies, and a couple/few more tablespoons of almond milk & enjoy with a good friend!

Homemade Vanilla Pudding

Ingredients

1/2 cup sugar

3 tablespoons cornstarch

2 cups organic dairy milk (2% or whole)

2 egg yolks

1 tablespoon unsalted butter

1 teaspoon vanilla extract

1 pinch salt

Directions

Whisk together the sugar, cornstarch, and salt in a saucepan.

Pour 1/4 cup of the milk into the sugar mixture, stirring to form a smooth paste. Whisk in the remaining milk and the egg yolks.

Cook the pudding mixture over low heat, stirring with a wooden spoon until thickened, about 10 minutes. Do not allow it to boil.

Remove from heat and stir in the butter and vanilla. Scrape the pudding into four individual bowls. (Unless making pudding cake; in that case, just scrape into a bowl.)

Cover each bowl with plastic wrap, pressing the surfaces to make an airtight seal. Refrigerate until well chilled, about 1 hour.

Tofu Scramble with Spinach and Tomatoes

Ingredients:

1 block of firm tofu, drained and crumbled

1 cup fresh spinach

1 cup cherry tomatoes, halved

1 tablespoon olive oil

1/2 teaspoon turmeric

Salt and pepper to taste

Optional: chopped fresh herbs like chives or parsley for garnish

Instructions:

Prepare the tofu: Heat olive oil in a pan over medium heat. Add crumbled tofu and cook for 2-3 minutes, stirring occasionally.

Add seasoning: Sprinkle turmeric over the tofu to give it a yellow color similar to scrambled eggs. Season with salt and pepper to taste.

Incorporate vegetables: Add cherry tomatoes to the pan and cook for another 2 minutes until they start to soften. Then, add fresh spinach and cook until it wilts, usually about 1-2 minutes.

Combine and cook: Mix everything together gently, ensuring the tofu and vegetables are evenly distributed. Cook for an additional 2-3 minutes to let the flavors meld.

Serve: Remove from heat and garnish with chopped fresh herbs if desired. Serve hot and enjoy!

How about a delicious smoothie bowl? Here's a low FODMAP, plant-based recipe for a Berry Smoothie Bowl:

Berry Smoothie Bowl

Ingredients:

1 cup mixed berries (blueberries, strawberries, raspberries)

1 ripe banana

1/2 cup lactose-free or almond milk

1 tablespoon chia seeds

Toppings: Sliced strawberries, blueberries, shredded coconut, sliced almonds (use FODMAP-friendly portions)

Instructions:

Prepare the base: In a blender, combine the mixed berries, banana, lactose-free or almond milk, and chia seeds. Blend until smooth and creamy.

Assemble the bowl: Pour the smoothie into a bowl.

Add toppings: Top the smoothie bowl with sliced strawberries, blueberries, shredded coconut, and sliced almonds (use FODMAP-friendly portions according to tolerance).

Quinoa Breakfast Bowl

Ingredients:

1 cup cooked quinoa

1/2 cup firm tofu, diced

1 cup spinach

1 small zucchini, sliced

1 tablespoon olive oil

1/2 teaspoon paprika

Salt and pepper to taste

Optional: Chopped fresh herbs like parsley or chives for garnish

Instructions:

Prepare the quinoa: Cook quinoa according to package instructions and set aside.

Cook the tofu and vegetables: In a pan, heat olive oil over medium heat. Add diced tofu and cook until slightly golden brown. Add sliced zucchini and cook for 2-3 minutes until tender. Add spinach and cook until wilted. Season with paprika, salt, and pepper.

Assemble the bowl: Place the cooked quinoa at the bottom of a bowl. Top it with the tofu, zucchini, and spinach mixture.

Garnish: Garnish with chopped fresh herbs like parsley or chives for added flavor.

Banana Almond Butter Toast

Ingredients:

2 slices of low FODMAP bread (such as sourdough or gluten-free bread)

2 tablespoons almond butter (check for no added high FODMAP ingredients)

1 ripe banana, sliced

Optional: A sprinkle of cinnamon or a drizzle of maple syrup (if tolerated)

Instructions:

Toast the bread: Toast the slices of bread to your desired level of doneness.

Spread almond butter: Once toasted, spread a generous layer of almond butter on each slice of bread.

Add banana slices: Arrange the banana slices on top of the almond butter layer.

Optional: Sprinkle a bit of cinnamon or drizzle a small amount of maple syrup over the bananas for extra flavor (if tolerated within your FODMAP limits).

Serve: Enjoy your delicious Banana Almond Butter Toast alongside a cup of herbal tea or your favorite low FODMAP beverage!

Low FODMAP Chia Seed Pudding with Berries

Ingredients:

2 tablespoons chia seeds

1 cup lactose-free or almond milk

1/2 teaspoon vanilla extract

1 tablespoon maple syrup (optional, if tolerated)

1/2 cup mixed low FODMAP berries (such as strawberries, blueberries, raspberries)

Sliced almonds (for topping, if tolerated)

Instructions:

Mix chia seeds and milk: In a bowl or a jar, combine chia seeds, lactose-free or almond milk, vanilla extract, and maple syrup (if using). Stir well to ensure the chia seeds are evenly distributed. Let it sit for a couple of minutes.

Stir again: After a few minutes, stir the mixture again to prevent clumping of chia seeds. Then, cover and refrigerate it overnight or for at least 2-3 hours until it thickens into a pudding-like consistency.

Prepare the toppings: Wash and slice the mixed berries. If tolerated, you can also lightly toast some sliced almonds for added crunch.

Assemble: Once the chia pudding has thickened, spoon it into a bowl. Top it with the mixed berries and sliced almonds.

Enjoy: Your delicious and nutritious Low FODMAP Chia Seed Pudding with Berries is ready to be enjoyed as a satisfying breakfast!

Spinach and Tomato Omelette

Ingredients:

2-3 large eggs (or your preferred egg substitute)

1 cup fresh spinach leaves, chopped

1/2 cup cherry tomatoes, halved

1 tablespoon olive oil

Salt and pepper to taste

Optional: Fresh herbs like basil or chives for garnish

Instructions:

Prepare the vegetables: Heat olive oil in a non-stick skillet over medium heat. Add the cherry tomatoes and cook for 1-2 minutes until they start to soften. Then, add the chopped spinach and sauté until wilted. Remove the vegetables from the pan and set them aside.

Whisk the eggs: In a bowl, whisk the eggs (or egg substitute) together until well combined. Season with salt and pepper.

Cook the omelette: Pour the whisked eggs into the skillet and swirl to ensure an even layer.

Allow the eggs to cook for a minute or so until they start setting at the edges.

Add vegetables: Once the edges of the omelette start to set, spread the cooked spinach and tomatoes over one half of the omelette.

Fold and finish cooking: Using a spatula, carefully fold the other half of the omelette over the vegetables. Let it cook for another minute until the eggs are fully set and the filling is warmed through.

Garnish and serve: Slide the omelette onto a plate, garnish with fresh herbs if desired, and enjoy a flavorful and protein-packed breakfast!

Low FODMAP Overnight Oats with Peanut Butter and Banana

Ingredients:

1/2 cup rolled oats (certified gluten-free if needed)

1 cup lactose-free or almond milk

1 tablespoon chia seeds

1 tablespoon natural peanut butter (check for no added high FODMAP ingredients)

1 ripe banana, sliced

Optional: A sprinkle of cinnamon

Instructions:

Combine ingredients: In a jar or bowl, mix together the rolled oats, lactose-free or almond milk, chia seeds, and peanut butter. Stir well to ensure all ingredients are combined.

Add banana slices: Gently fold in the sliced banana into the oat mixture.

Cover and refrigerate: Cover the jar or bowl and refrigerate it overnight or for at least 4 hours to allow the oats and chia seeds to absorb the liquid and soften.

Optional: Before serving, sprinkle a bit of cinnamon for added flavor if desired.

Enjoy: Your delicious and creamy Low FODMAP Overnight Oats with Peanut Butter and Banana are ready to be enjoyed straight from the fridge in the morning!

Low FODMAP Blueberry Banana Pancakes

Ingredients:

1 ripe banana, mashed

1 cup gluten-free flour (such as rice flour or oat flour)

1 teaspoon baking powder (check for no added high FODMAP ingredients)

1/2 cup lactose-free or almond milk

1/2 cup blueberries

1 tablespoon maple syrup (optional, if tolerated)

Cooking oil or cooking spray for the pan

Instructions:

Prepare the batter: In a mixing bowl, mash the ripe banana. Add the gluten-free flour, baking powder, lactose-free or almond milk, and maple syrup (if using). Mix until a smooth batter forms.

Fold in blueberries: Gently fold in the blueberries into the pancake batter.

Heat the pan: Heat a non-stick skillet or griddle over medium heat. Lightly grease the surface with cooking oil or cooking spray.

Cook the pancakes: Pour small portions of the batter onto the heated skillet to form pancakes.

Cook until bubbles form on the surface, then flip and cook until golden brown on both sides.

Serve: Stack the pancakes on a plate and top with extra blueberries or a drizzle of maple syrup if desired.

Tofu Breakfast Burrito

Ingredients:

1 block firm tofu, drained and crumbled

1 tablespoon olive oil

1 teaspoon turmeric

1/2 teaspoon smoked paprika

Salt and pepper to taste

1 cup spinach

1/2 cup diced tomatoes (canned or fresh)

2-3 gluten-free tortillas (check for low FODMAP ingredients)

Optional toppings:

Sliced avocado

Low FODMAP salsa

Chopped fresh cilantro

Lactose-free cheese (if tolerated)

Instructions:

Prepare the tofu scramble: Heat olive oil in a skillet over medium heat. Add crumbled tofu, turmeric, smoked paprika, salt, and pepper. Cook for 5-7 minutes until the tofu starts to brown slightly.

Add vegetables: Add diced tomatoes and spinach to the skillet with the tofu. Cook for an additional 2-3 minutes until the spinach wilts and the tomatoes soften.

Warm the tortillas: Heat the gluten-free tortillas in a separate skillet or microwave for a few seconds to make them pliable.

Assemble the burritos: Spoon the tofu and vegetable mixture onto the center of each warmed tortilla. Add optional toppings like sliced avocado, low FODMAP salsa, chopped fresh cilantro, or lactose-free cheese if desired.

Roll the burritos: Fold the sides of the tortilla over the filling, then roll it up tightly to create a burrito.

Serve: Slice the burritos in half and serve them warm. They're a protein-packed and satisfying breakfast option that's easy to customize with your favorite low FODMAP toppings!

LUNCH LOW-FODMAP DIET RECIPES

Quinoa Salad with Roasted Vegetables

Ingredients:

1 cup quinoa, rinsed

2 cups low FODMAP vegetable broth or water

2 cups mixed low FODMAP vegetables (bell peppers, zucchini, carrots, etc.), chopped

2 tablespoons olive oil

Salt and pepper to taste

1 tablespoon fresh lemon juice

2 tablespoons chopped fresh herbs (such as parsley or chives)

Instructions:

Preheat oven and prepare vegetables: Preheat your oven to 400°F (200°C). Toss the chopped vegetables with 1 tablespoon of olive oil, salt, and pepper. Spread them on a baking sheet and roast for 20-25 minutes or until they're tender and slightly caramelized.

Cook quinoa: While the vegetables are roasting, cook the quinoa. Rinse the quinoa under cold water and then combine it with the low FODMAP vegetable broth or water in a saucepan. Bring to a boil, then reduce heat to low, cover, and simmer for 15-20 minutes or until the quinoa is cooked and the liquid is absorbed.

Assemble the salad: In a large mixing bowl, combine the cooked quinoa and roasted vegetables. Add the remaining olive oil, fresh lemon juice, and chopped herbs. Toss everything together gently until well combined.

Adjust seasoning and serve: Taste the salad and adjust the seasoning if needed with more salt, pepper, or lemon juice. Serve the quinoa salad warm or at room temperature.

Vegetable Stir-Fry with Tofu

Ingredients:

1 block firm tofu, drained and cubed

2 tablespoons garlic-infused oil (for low FODMAP option)

2 cups mixed low FODMAP vegetables (bell peppers, bok choy, carrots, snow peas, etc.), sliced

1-inch piece of fresh ginger, grated

2 tablespoons low-sodium soy sauce (for gluten-free, ensure it's low FODMAP)

Salt and pepper to taste

Optional: Chopped green onions (green parts only, for those who tolerate them)

Instructions:

Prepare the tofu: Heat 1 tablespoon of garlic-infused oil in a large skillet or wok over medium heat. Add the cubed tofu and cook until golden brown on all sides, stirring occasionally. Remove the tofu from the skillet and set it aside.

Stir-fry the vegetables: In the same skillet, add the remaining garlic-infused oil if needed. Add the mixed vegetables and grated ginger. Stir-fry for 3-4 minutes until the vegetables are tender-crisp.

Add tofu and seasoning: Return the cooked tofu to the skillet with the vegetables. Pour in the low-sodium soy sauce. Season with salt and pepper to taste. Toss everything together until well combined.

Optional: If using, sprinkle chopped green onions over the stir-fry for added flavor.

Serve: Transfer the Vegetable Stir-Fry with Tofu to a serving dish and enjoy this flavorful and protein-rich plant-based lunch!

Mediterranean Quinoa Salad

Ingredients:

1 cup quinoa, rinsed

2 cups low FODMAP vegetable broth or water

1 cup cherry tomatoes, halved

1 cucumber, diced

1/2 cup chopped red bell pepper

1/4 cup chopped Kalamata olives (check for no added high FODMAP ingredients)

1/4 cup chopped fresh parsley

2 tablespoons olive oil

2 tablespoons fresh lemon juice

Salt and pepper to taste

Instructions:

Cook quinoa: In a saucepan, combine the rinsed quinoa and low FODMAP vegetable broth or water. Bring to a boil, then reduce heat to low, cover, and simmer for 15-20 minutes or until the quinoa is cooked and the liquid is absorbed. Let it cool.

Prepare vegetables: In a large bowl, combine the cooked quinoa, cherry tomatoes, diced cucumber, chopped red bell pepper, chopped Kalamata olives, and chopped fresh parsley.

Dress the salad: Drizzle olive oil and fresh lemon juice over the salad. Season with salt and pepper to taste. Toss everything gently until well combined.

Chill and serve: Refrigerate the salad for at least 30 minutes to allow the flavors to meld together. Serve the chilled Low FODMAP Mediterranean

Quinoa Salad as a refreshing and nutritious lunch option!

Veggie and Tofu Rice Paper Rolls

Ingredients:

Rice paper wrappers (check for low FODMAP ingredients)

1 block firm tofu, drained and cut into thin strips

1 cup mixed low FODMAP vegetables (lettuce, carrots, bell peppers, cucumber), julienned

Fresh herbs like cilantro or mint leaves

Low FODMAP dipping sauce (such as a combination of tamari, sesame oil, and a touch of maple syrup)

Instructions:

Prepare the tofu: Heat a non-stick skillet over medium heat. Add a little oil and cook the tofu strips until they're golden brown on both sides. Remove from heat and set aside.

Prepare the vegetables and herbs: Julienne the mixed vegetables and set them aside. Wash and prepare the fresh herbs.

Soften rice paper wrappers: Fill a large shallow dish or bowl with warm water. Dip one rice paper wrapper into the warm water for about 15-20 seconds until it softens. Place it on a clean, damp kitchen towel or a plate.

Assemble the rolls: Place a few strips of tofu, a handful of julienned vegetables, and some fresh herbs (cilantro or mint leaves) in the center of the softened rice paper wrapper, leaving some space on the sides. Fold the sides of the wrapper over the filling, then tightly roll it up from the bottom to enclose the filling.

Repeat and serve: Continue assembling the rolls with the remaining ingredients. Serve the Low

FODMAP Veggie and Tofu Rice Paper Rolls with the low FODMAP dipping sauce.

Quinoa Stuffed Bell Peppers

Ingredients:

4 bell peppers (red, yellow, or green)

1 cup quinoa, rinsed

2 cups low FODMAP vegetable broth or water

1 tablespoon olive oil

1 cup mixed low FODMAP vegetables (such as zucchini, carrots, spinach), diced

1/2 cup diced tomatoes (canned or fresh)

1 teaspoon dried oregano

Salt and pepper to taste

Optional: Grated lactose-free cheese (if tolerated)

Instructions:

Prepare the bell peppers: Preheat the oven to 375°F (190°C). Cut the tops off the bell peppers and remove the seeds and membranes from the insides. Place the bell peppers in a baking dish, cut-side up.

Cook quinoa: In a saucepan, combine the rinsed quinoa and low FODMAP vegetable broth or water. Bring to a boil, then reduce heat to low, cover, and simmer for 15-20 minutes or until the quinoa is cooked and the liquid is absorbed.

Prepare the filling: In a skillet, heat olive oil over medium heat. Add the diced mixed vegetables and sauté for a few minutes until they start to soften. Add the diced tomatoes, dried oregano, salt, and pepper. Cook for an additional 2-3 minutes.

Combine quinoa and filling: In a mixing bowl, combine the cooked quinoa with the sautéed vegetable mixture. Mix well to combine all the flavors.

Stuff the bell peppers: Spoon the quinoa and vegetable mixture into the hollowed-out bell peppers, packing it gently. If desired, top each stuffed bell pepper with a sprinkle of grated lactose-free cheese.

Bake: Cover the baking dish with foil and bake in the preheated oven for 25-30 minutes, or until the bell peppers are tender.

Serve: Remove from the oven and let them cool slightly before serving. Enjoy these flavorful and satisfying Low FODMAP Quinoa Stuffed Bell Peppers!

Tofu and Veggie Stir-Fry with Brown Rice

Ingredients:

1 block firm tofu, drained and cubed

2 tablespoons garlic-infused oil (for low FODMAP option)

2 cups mixed low FODMAP vegetables (bell peppers, bok choy, carrots, snow peas, etc.), sliced

1-inch piece of fresh ginger, grated

2 tablespoons low-sodium soy sauce (for gluten-free, ensure it's low FODMAP)

Salt and pepper to taste

2 cups cooked brown rice

Instructions:

Prepare the tofu: Heat 1 tablespoon of garlic-infused oil in a large skillet or wok over medium heat. Add the cubed tofu and cook until golden brown on all sides, stirring occasionally. Remove the tofu from the skillet and set it aside.

Stir-fry the vegetables: In the same skillet, add the remaining garlic-infused oil if needed. Add the mixed vegetables and grated ginger. Stir-fry for 3-4 minutes until the vegetables are tender-crisp.

Add tofu and seasoning: Return the cooked tofu to the skillet with the vegetables. Pour in the low-sodium soy sauce. Season with salt and pepper to taste. Toss everything together until well combined.

Serve: Divide the cooked brown rice into serving bowls or plates. Top with the Tofu and Veggie Stir-Fry mixture.

Quinoa and Chickpea Salad

Ingredients:

1 cup quinoa, rinsed

2 cups low FODMAP vegetable broth or water

1 can (15 oz) chickpeas, drained and rinsed

1 cup mixed low FODMAP vegetables (cucumbers, tomatoes, bell peppers), diced

2 tablespoons chopped fresh parsley

2 tablespoons olive oil

2 tablespoons fresh lemon juice

Salt and pepper to taste

Instructions:

Cook quinoa: In a saucepan, combine the rinsed quinoa and low FODMAP vegetable broth or water. Bring to a boil, then reduce heat to low, cover, and simmer for 15-20 minutes or until the quinoa is cooked and the liquid is absorbed. Allow it to cool.

Prepare chickpeas and vegetables: In a large bowl, combine the cooked quinoa, chickpeas, diced mixed vegetables, and chopped fresh parsley.

Make dressing: In a small bowl, whisk together the olive oil and fresh lemon juice. Season with salt and pepper to taste.

Assemble salad: Pour the dressing over the quinoa, chickpea, and vegetable mixture. Toss everything gently until well combined.

Chill and serve: Refrigerate the salad for at least 30 minutes before serving to allow the flavors to meld. Enjoy the Low FODMAP Quinoa and Chickpea Salad as a refreshing and nutritious lunch!

Lentil and Vegetable Soup

Ingredients:

1 cup dried green or brown lentils, rinsed

6 cups low FODMAP vegetable broth

1 cup diced carrots

1 cup diced zucchini

1 cup diced bell peppers (red, yellow, or green)

1 cup diced tomatoes (canned or fresh)

1 tablespoon garlic-infused oil (for low FODMAP option)

1 teaspoon dried thyme

Salt and pepper to taste

Fresh chopped parsley for garnish (optional)

Instructions:

Cook lentils: In a large pot, combine the rinsed lentils and low FODMAP vegetable broth. Bring to a boil, then reduce heat to a simmer. Cook for about 15-20 minutes or until the lentils are tender but not mushy.

Prepare vegetables: In a separate skillet, heat the garlic-infused oil over medium heat. Add the diced carrots, zucchini, bell peppers, and cook for 5-7 minutes until they start to soften.

Combine vegetables and lentils: Add the sautéed vegetables to the pot of cooked lentils. Stir in the diced tomatoes and dried thyme. Simmer for an additional 10-15 minutes to let the flavors meld together.

Season and serve: Season the soup with salt and pepper to taste. Ladle the Low FODMAP Lentil and Vegetable Soup into bowls. Optionally, garnish with fresh chopped parsley for added flavor.

Tofu Buddha Bowl

Ingredients:

1 block firm tofu, drained and cubed

2 tablespoons garlic-infused oil (for low FODMAP option)

2 cups mixed greens (lettuce, spinach, arugula, etc.)

1 cup cooked quinoa or rice

1/2 cup shredded carrots

1/2 cup sliced cucumber

1/2 cup diced bell peppers (red, yellow, or green)

1/4 cup sliced radishes

1/4 cup chopped green tops of green onions (for those who tolerate them)

2 tablespoons sesame seeds (optional)

Low FODMAP dressing (such as a mix of olive oil, rice vinegar, and a touch of maple syrup)

Instructions:

Prepare the tofu: Heat 1 tablespoon of garlic-infused oil in a skillet over medium heat. Add the cubed tofu and cook until golden brown on all sides. Remove from heat and set aside.

Assemble the bowl: Divide the mixed greens, cooked quinoa or rice, shredded carrots, sliced cucumber, diced bell peppers, and sliced radishes into serving bowls.

Add tofu and toppings: Top the bowls with the cooked tofu cubes. If using, sprinkle the chopped green tops of green onions and sesame seeds over the bowls.

Drizzle dressing: Drizzle the Low FODMAP dressing over the Buddha bowls just before serving.

Mediterranean Quinoa Salad Wrap

Ingredients:

1 cup cooked quinoa

1/2 cup diced tomatoes (canned or fresh)

1/4 cup chopped cucumber

1/4 cup chopped red bell pepper

2 tablespoons chopped Kalamata olives (check for no added high FODMAP ingredients)

2 tablespoons chopped fresh parsley

1 tablespoon olive oil

1 tablespoon fresh lemon juice

Salt and pepper to taste

Low FODMAP wrap or tortilla (check for low FODMAP ingredients)

Mixed greens or lettuce leaves

Instructions:

Prepare the quinoa salad: In a bowl, combine the cooked quinoa, diced tomatoes, chopped cucumber, chopped red bell pepper, chopped Kalamata olives, chopped fresh parsley, olive oil, and fresh lemon juice. Season with salt and pepper to taste. Mix well.

Assemble the wrap: Lay a low FODMAP wrap or tortilla on a clean surface. Place a few mixed greens or lettuce leaves on the wrap.

Add quinoa salad: Spoon the prepared Mediterranean quinoa salad onto the greens in the center of the wrap.

Fold and roll: Fold in the sides of the wrap, then roll it up tightly from the bottom to enclose the filling, creating a wrap.

Slice and serve: Carefully slice the wrap in half if desired, and serve immediately.

Sushi Bowl

Ingredients:

1 cup cooked sushi rice (or substitute with quinoa for a different twist)

1/2 cup sliced cucumber

1/2 cup sliced red bell pepper

1/2 cup sliced carrots

1/2 cup sliced radishes

1/2 cup diced firm tofu

1 tablespoon sesame seeds (optional)

2 tablespoons low-sodium soy sauce (for gluten-free, ensure it's low FODMAP)

1 tablespoon rice vinegar

1 tablespoon maple syrup

1 teaspoon sesame oil

Nori strips (seaweed sheets), sliced into thin strips for garnish (optional)

Instructions:

Prepare the dressing: In a small bowl, whisk together the low-sodium soy sauce, rice vinegar, maple syrup, and sesame oil. Set aside.

Assemble the bowl: Divide the cooked sushi rice or quinoa into serving bowls. Arrange the sliced cucumber, red bell pepper, carrots, radishes, and diced tofu on top of the rice in separate sections.

Drizzle the dressing: Drizzle the prepared dressing over the ingredients in the bowl. Sprinkle sesame seeds on top if using.

Garnish with nori strips: If desired, garnish the bowls with sliced nori strips for added flavor.

Mexican Quinoa Bowl

Ingredients:

1 cup cooked quinoa

1 cup diced tomatoes (canned or fresh)

1 cup cooked and drained black beans (canned, rinsed)

1/2 cup sliced bell peppers (red, yellow, or green)

1/2 cup sliced cucumber

1/4 cup chopped fresh cilantro

2 tablespoons sliced black olives (check for no added high FODMAP ingredients)

1 tablespoon olive oil

1 tablespoon fresh lime juice

1 teaspoon ground cumin

Salt and pepper to taste

Optional: Sliced jalapeños (if tolerated)

Instructions:

Prepare the quinoa: Cook quinoa according to package instructions and set aside.

Prepare the vegetables and beans: In a bowl, combine the diced tomatoes, cooked black beans, sliced bell peppers, sliced cucumber, chopped fresh cilantro, and sliced black olives.

Make the dressing: In a small bowl, whisk together the olive oil, fresh lime juice, ground cumin, salt, and pepper.

Assemble the bowl: Divide the cooked quinoa into serving bowls. Top with the prepared vegetable and bean mixture.

Drizzle with dressing: Drizzle the dressing over the ingredients in the bowl.

Optional: If desired, add sliced jalapeños for a bit of heat.

Veggie Stir-Fry Noodle Bowl

Ingredients:

8 oz (about 225g) rice noodles (check for low FODMAP ingredients)

2 tablespoons garlic-infused oil (for low FODMAP option)

1 block firm tofu, drained and cubed

2 cups mixed low FODMAP vegetables (bell peppers, carrots, bok choy, etc.), sliced

1 tablespoon low-sodium soy sauce (for gluten-free, ensure it's low FODMAP)

1 tablespoon rice vinegar

1 tablespoon maple syrup

Sesame seeds for garnish (optional)

Chopped green tops of green onions (for those who tolerate them) for garnish (optional)

Instructions:

Prepare the rice noodles: Cook the rice noodles according to package instructions. Drain and set aside.

Cook the tofu: Heat 1 tablespoon of garlic-infused oil in a large skillet or wok over medium heat. Add the cubed tofu and cook until golden brown on all sides. Remove the tofu from the skillet and set it aside.

Stir-fry the vegetables: In the same skillet, add the remaining tablespoon of garlic-infused oil if needed. Add the mixed vegetables and stir-fry for 3-4 minutes until they are tender-crisp.

Combine tofu and vegetables: Return the cooked tofu to the skillet with the vegetables.

Make the sauce: In a small bowl, whisk together the low-sodium soy sauce, rice vinegar, and maple syrup. Pour the sauce over the tofu and vegetables in the skillet. Toss everything together until well coated and heated through.

Assemble the noodle bowls: Divide the cooked rice noodles into serving bowls. Top with the tofu and vegetable stir-fry.

Garnish and serve: Garnish with sesame seeds and chopped green tops of green onions if using.

Quinoa and Roasted Vegetable Salad

Ingredients:

1 cup quinoa, rinsed

2 cups low FODMAP vegetable broth or water

2 cups mixed low FODMAP vegetables (bell peppers, zucchini, carrots, eggplant), diced

2 tablespoons olive oil

Salt and pepper to taste

1 tablespoon fresh lemon juice

2 tablespoons chopped fresh parsley

Optional: Feta cheese (if tolerated)

Instructions:

Prepare the quinoa: In a saucepan, combine the rinsed quinoa and low FODMAP vegetable broth or water. Bring to a boil, then reduce heat to low, cover, and simmer for 15-20 minutes or until the quinoa is cooked and the liquid is absorbed. Set aside.

Roast the vegetables: Preheat the oven to 400°F (200°C). Toss the diced mixed vegetables with olive oil, salt, and pepper. Spread them on a baking sheet and roast for about 20-25 minutes or until they're tender and slightly caramelized.

Remove from the oven and let them cool slightly.

Assemble the salad: In a large mixing bowl, combine the cooked quinoa and roasted vegetables. Add fresh lemon juice and chopped parsley. Toss gently until well mixed.

Optional: If desired and tolerated, crumble feta cheese on top of the salad for added flavor.

Serve: This Low FODMAP Quinoa and Roasted Vegetable Salad can be served warm or at room temperature. It's a hearty and flavorful lunch option that's packed with nutrients and customizable with your favorite low FODMAP veggies!

Thai Peanut Tofu Bowl

Ingredients:

1 block firm tofu, drained and cubed

2 tablespoons garlic-infused oil (for low FODMAP option)

1 cup cooked rice or quinoa

2 cups mixed low FODMAP vegetables (bell peppers, carrots, zucchini), sliced

1/4 cup chopped peanuts (check for no added high FODMAP ingredients)

Fresh cilantro for garnish

Lime wedges for serving

For the peanut sauce:

2 tablespoons peanut butter (ensure no high FODMAP ingredients)

2 tablespoons low-sodium soy sauce (for gluten-free, ensure it's low FODMAP)

1 tablespoon maple syrup

1 tablespoon rice vinegar

1 teaspoon sesame oil

Water (to adjust consistency)

Instructions:

Prepare the peanut sauce: In a small bowl, whisk together the peanut butter, low-sodium soy sauce, maple syrup, rice vinegar, and sesame oil. Add water gradually to reach the desired consistency. Set aside.

Cook the tofu: Heat 1 tablespoon of garlic-infused oil in a skillet over medium heat. Add the cubed tofu and cook until golden brown on all sides. Remove the tofu from the skillet and set it aside.

Stir-fry the vegetables: In the same skillet, add the remaining tablespoon of garlic-infused oil if needed. Stir-fry the mixed vegetables for 3-4 minutes until they are tender-crisp.

Assemble the bowl: Divide the cooked rice or quinoa into serving bowls. Top with the stir-fried vegetables and cooked tofu.

Drizzle with peanut sauce: Drizzle the prepared peanut sauce over the ingredients in the bowl.

Garnish and serve: Garnish with chopped peanuts, fresh cilantro, and serve with lime wedges on the side.

Eggplant and Zucchini Ratatouille

Ingredients:

1 large eggplant, diced

2 medium zucchinis, diced

1 red bell pepper, diced

1 yellow bell pepper, diced

1 can (14 oz) diced tomatoes (check for no high
FODMAP ingredients)

2 tablespoons garlic-infused oil (for low FODMAP option)

1 teaspoon dried thyme

1 teaspoon dried oregano

Salt and pepper to taste

Fresh basil leaves for garnish

Instructions:

Preheat the oven: Preheat your oven to 375°F (190°C).

Prepare the vegetables: In a large bowl, combine the diced eggplant, zucchinis, red bell pepper, yellow bell pepper, diced tomatoes, garlic-infused oil, dried thyme, dried oregano, salt, and pepper. Mix well until the vegetables are evenly coated.

Bake the ratatouille: Transfer the vegetable mixture to a baking dish. Spread it out evenly. Cover the dish with foil and bake for about 45-50 minutes or until the vegetables are tender.

Garnish and serve: Once cooked, remove from the oven. Garnish the Low FODMAP Eggplant and Zucchini Ratatouille with fresh basil leaves before serving.

Lentil Soup

Ingredients:

1 cup dried green or brown lentils, rinsed

6 cups low FODMAP vegetable broth

2 medium carrots, diced

2 stalks celery, diced

1 medium potato, diced

1 teaspoon dried thyme

1 bay leaf

2 tablespoons garlic-infused oil (for low FODMAP option)

Salt and pepper to taste

Fresh parsley for garnish

Instructions:

Prepare lentils and vegetables: Rinse the lentils under cold water and set them aside. In a large pot, heat the garlic-infused oil over medium heat. Add diced carrots, celery, and potato. Sauté for about 5 minutes until slightly softened.

Cook the soup: Add the rinsed lentils, dried thyme, bay leaf, and low FODMAP vegetable broth to the pot. Bring the mixture to a boil, then reduce heat to a simmer. Cover and let it simmer for 25-30 minutes or until the lentils and vegetables are tender.

Season and serve: Once the soup is cooked, season with salt and pepper to taste. Remove the bay leaf.

Garnish and serve: Ladle the Low FODMAP Lentil Soup into bowls and garnish with fresh chopped parsley.

Stir-Fried Ginger Beef with Vegetables

Ingredients:

1 pound (450g) beef sirloin or flank steak, thinly sliced

2 tablespoons garlic-infused oil (for low FODMAP option)

1 tablespoon freshly grated ginger

2 cups mixed low FODMAP vegetables (bell peppers, carrots, bok choy, etc.), sliced

2 tablespoons low-sodium soy sauce (for gluten-free, ensure it's low FODMAP)

1 tablespoon rice vinegar

Salt and pepper to taste

Cooked rice or quinoa for serving

Instructions:

Marinate the beef: In a bowl, mix the thinly sliced beef with freshly grated ginger. Let it marinate for about 15-20 minutes.

Stir-fry the beef: Heat 1 tablespoon of garlic-infused oil in a large skillet or wok over high heat. Add the marinated beef and stir-fry for 2-3 minutes until it's browned. Remove the beef from the skillet and set it aside.

Cook the vegetables: In the same skillet, add the remaining tablespoon of garlic-infused oil if needed. Add the mixed vegetables and stir-fry for 3-4 minutes until they are tender-crisp.

Combine beef and vegetables: Return the cooked beef to the skillet with the vegetables.

Make the sauce: In a small bowl, mix together the low-sodium soy sauce and rice vinegar. Pour the sauce over the beef and vegetables in the skillet. Toss everything together until well coated and heated through.

Serve: Serve the Stir-Fried Ginger Beef and Vegetables over cooked rice or quinoa.

Quinoa and Roasted Vegetable Bowl

Ingredients:

1 cup quinoa, rinsed

2 cups low FODMAP vegetable broth or water

2 cups mixed low FODMAP vegetables (bell peppers, zucchini, carrots, eggplant), diced

2 tablespoons olive oil

Salt and pepper to taste

1 tablespoon fresh lemon juice

2 tablespoons chopped fresh parsley

Optional: Feta cheese (if tolerated)

Instructions:

Prepare the quinoa: In a saucepan, combine the rinsed quinoa and low FODMAP vegetable broth or water. Bring to a boil, then reduce heat to low, cover, and simmer for 15-20 minutes or until the quinoa is cooked and the liquid is absorbed. Set aside.

Roast the vegetables: Preheat the oven to 400°F (200°C). Toss the diced mixed vegetables with olive oil, salt, and pepper. Spread them on a baking sheet and roast for about 20-25 minutes or until they're tender and slightly caramelized. Remove from the oven and let them cool slightly.

Assemble the bowl: In a large mixing bowl, combine the cooked quinoa and roasted vegetables. Add fresh lemon juice and chopped parsley. Toss gently until well mixed.

Optional: If desired and tolerated, crumble feta cheese on top of the bowl for added flavor.

Serve: This Quinoa and Roasted Vegetable Bowl can be served warm or at room temperature. It's a hearty and flavorful dinner option that's packed with nutrients and customizable with your favorite low FODMAP veggies!

Veggie Stir-Fry with Tofu

Ingredients:

1 block firm tofu, drained and cubed

2 tablespoons garlic-infused oil (for low FODMAP option)

2 cups mixed low FODMAP vegetables (bell peppers, carrots, bok choy, etc.), sliced

1 tablespoon low-sodium soy sauce (for gluten-free, ensure it's low FODMAP)

1 tablespoon rice vinegar

1 tablespoon maple syrup

Sesame seeds for garnish (optional)

Cooked rice or quinoa for serving

Instructions:

Prepare the tofu: Heat 1 tablespoon of garlic-infused oil in a skillet over medium heat. Add the cubed tofu and cook until golden brown on all sides. Remove the tofu from the skillet and set it aside.

Stir-fry the vegetables: In the same skillet, add the remaining tablespoon of garlic-infused oil if needed. Stir-fry the mixed vegetables for 3-4 minutes until they are tender-crisp.

Combine tofu and vegetables: Return the cooked tofu to the skillet with the vegetables.

Make the sauce: In a small bowl, whisk together the low-sodium soy sauce, rice vinegar, and maple syrup. Pour the sauce over the tofu and vegetables in the skillet. Toss everything together until well coated and heated through.

Serve: Serve the Veggie Stir-Fry with Tofu over cooked rice or quinoa. Garnish with sesame seeds if desired.

Mediterranean Stuffed Peppers

Ingredients:

4 bell peppers (red, yellow, or green)

1 cup cooked quinoa

1 cup diced tomatoes (canned or fresh)

1 cup diced zucchini

1 cup diced eggplant

1/4 cup chopped fresh parsley

2 tablespoons olive oil

1 teaspoon dried oregano

Salt and pepper to taste

Instructions:

Prepare the peppers: Preheat the oven to 375°F (190°C). Cut the tops off the bell peppers and remove the seeds and membranes. Place the peppers in a baking dish.

Prepare the filling: In a skillet, heat olive oil over medium heat. Add diced zucchini, eggplant, and tomatoes. Cook for about 5 minutes until slightly softened. Add cooked quinoa, dried oregano, salt, pepper, and chopped parsley. Stir well to combine.

Stuff the peppers: Spoon the quinoa and vegetable mixture into the hollowed-out bell peppers, packing it gently.

Bake: Cover the baking dish with foil and bake for 30-35 minutes or until the peppers are tender.

Serve: Remove from the oven and let them cool slightly before serving. These Mediterranean Stuffed Peppers are a delightful and satisfying dinner option.

Tofu and Vegetable Stir-Fry

Ingredients:

1 block firm tofu, drained and cubed

2 tablespoons garlic-infused oil (for low FODMAP option)

2 cups mixed low FODMAP vegetables (bell peppers, carrots, bok choy, etc.), sliced

1 tablespoon low-sodium soy sauce (for gluten-free, ensure it's low FODMAP)

1 tablespoon rice vinegar

1 tablespoon maple syrup

Sesame seeds for garnish (optional)

Cooked rice or quinoa for serving

Instructions:

Prepare the tofu: Heat 1 tablespoon of garlic-infused oil in a skillet over medium heat. Add the cubed tofu and cook until golden brown on all sides. Remove the tofu from the skillet and set it aside.

Stir-fry the vegetables: In the same skillet, add the remaining tablespoon of garlic-infused oil if needed. Stir-fry the mixed vegetables for 3-4 minutes until they are tender-crisp.

Combine tofu and vegetables: Return the cooked tofu to the skillet with the vegetables.

Make the sauce: In a small bowl, mix together the low-sodium soy sauce, rice vinegar, and maple syrup. Pour the sauce over the tofu and vegetables in the skillet. Toss everything together until well coated and heated through.

Serve: Serve the Stir-Fried Tofu and Vegetables over cooked rice or quinoa. Garnish with sesame seeds if desired.

Veggie and Tofu Stir-Fry

Ingredients:

1 block firm tofu, drained and cubed

2 tablespoons garlic-infused oil (for low FODMAP option)

2 cups mixed low FODMAP vegetables (bell peppers, carrots, zucchini), sliced

1 tablespoon low-sodium soy sauce (for gluten-free, ensure it's low FODMAP)

1 tablespoon rice vinegar

1 tablespoon maple syrup

Cooked rice or quinoa for serving

Instructions:

Prepare the tofu: Heat 1 tablespoon of garlic-infused oil in a skillet over medium heat. Add the cubed tofu and cook until golden brown on all sides. Remove the tofu from the skillet and set aside.

Stir-fry the vegetables: In the same skillet, add the remaining tablespoon of garlic-infused oil if needed. Stir-fry the mixed vegetables for 3-4 minutes until they are tender-crisp.

Combine tofu and vegetables: Return the cooked tofu to the skillet with the vegetables.

Make the sauce: In a small bowl, mix together the low-sodium soy sauce, rice vinegar, and maple syrup. Pour the sauce over the tofu and vegetables in the skillet. Toss everything together until well coated and heated through.

Serve: Serve the Veggie and Tofu Stir-Fry over cooked rice or quinoa.

Mexican Quinoa Bowl

Ingredients:

1 cup quinoa, rinsed

2 cups low FODMAP vegetable broth or water

1 cup diced tomatoes (canned or fresh)

1 cup cooked and drained black beans (canned, rinsed)

1/2 cup sliced bell peppers (red, yellow, or green)

1/2 cup sliced cucumber

1/4 cup chopped fresh cilantro

2 tablespoons sliced black olives (check for no added high FODMAP ingredients)

1 tablespoon olive oil

1 tablespoon fresh lime juice

1 teaspoon ground cumin

Salt and pepper to taste

Instructions:

Prepare the quinoa: Cook quinoa according to package instructions using low FODMAP vegetable broth or water. Set aside.

Prepare the vegetables: In a bowl, combine diced tomatoes, black beans, sliced bell peppers, sliced cucumber, chopped fresh cilantro, and sliced black olives.

Make the dressing: In a small bowl, whisk together olive oil, fresh lime juice, ground cumin, salt, and pepper.

Assemble the bowl: Divide the cooked quinoa into serving bowls. Top with the prepared vegetable and bean mixture.

Drizzle with dressing: Drizzle the dressing over the ingredients in the bowl.

Lentil and Spinach Curry

Ingredients:

1 cup dried lentils, rinsed

4 cups low FODMAP vegetable broth

1 tablespoon garlic-infused oil (for low FODMAP option)

1 cup diced tomatoes (canned or fresh)

2 cups fresh spinach

1 teaspoon ground cumin

1 teaspoon ground coriander

1 teaspoon turmeric

1/2 teaspoon paprika

Salt and pepper to taste

Cooked rice for serving

Instructions:

Cook the lentils: In a pot, combine the rinsed lentils and low FODMAP vegetable broth. Bring to a boil, then reduce heat to a simmer. Cook for 20-25 minutes or until the lentils are tender.

Prepare the curry: In a separate large skillet, heat garlic-infused oil over medium heat. Add diced tomatoes, ground cumin, ground coriander, turmeric, paprika, salt, and pepper. Cook for a few minutes until the tomatoes soften.

Combine ingredients: Add the cooked lentils (with any remaining broth) to the skillet with the tomato mixture. Stir well to combine. Add fresh spinach and continue to cook for another 3-4 minutes until the spinach wilts.

Serve: Serve the lentil and spinach curry over cooked rice.

Eggplant & Tofu Stir-Fry

Ingredients:

1 large eggplant, diced

1 block firm tofu, drained and cubed

2 tablespoons garlic-infused oil (for low FODMAP option)

2 cups mixed low FODMAP vegetables (bell peppers, carrots, bok choy), sliced

1 tablespoon low-sodium soy sauce (for gluten-free, ensure it's low FODMAP)

1 tablespoon rice vinegar

1 tablespoon maple syrup

Cooked rice or quinoa for serving

Instructions:

Prepare the eggplant: Place the diced eggplant in a colander and sprinkle it with salt. Let it sit for 20-30 minutes to draw out excess moisture. Rinse and pat dry.

Prepare the tofu: Heat 1 tablespoon of garlic-infused oil in a skillet over medium heat. Add the cubed tofu and cook until golden brown on all sides. Remove the tofu from the skillet and set it aside.

Stir-fry the vegetables: In the same skillet, add the remaining tablespoon of garlic-infused oil if needed. Add the mixed vegetables and diced eggplant. Stir-fry for 5-7 minutes until they are tender.

Combine tofu and vegetables: Return the cooked tofu to the skillet with the vegetables.

Make the sauce: In a small bowl, mix together the low-sodium soy sauce, rice vinegar, and maple syrup. Pour the sauce over the tofu and vegetables in the skillet. Toss everything together until well coated and heated through.

Serve: Serve the Eggplant & Tofu Stir-Fry over cooked rice or quinoa.

Low FODMAP Lentil and Vegetable Soup

Ingredients:

1 cup dried green lentils, rinsed

4 cups low FODMAP vegetable broth

1 cup diced carrots

1 cup diced zucchini

1 cup diced potatoes

1 cup chopped spinach

1 tablespoon garlic-infused oil (for low FODMAP option)

1 teaspoon dried thyme

1 teaspoon dried oregano

Salt and pepper to taste

Fresh parsley for garnish

Instructions:

Cook the lentils: In a pot, combine the rinsed lentils and low FODMAP vegetable broth. Bring to a boil, then reduce heat to a simmer. Cook for about 20-25 minutes or until the lentils are tender.

Prepare the vegetables: In a separate skillet, heat garlic-infused oil over medium heat. Add diced carrots, zucchini, potatoes, and cook for about 5 minutes until slightly softened.

Combine ingredients: Add the cooked vegetables to the pot with the lentils. Stir in dried thyme, dried oregano, salt, and pepper. Simmer for an additional 10-15 minutes.

Add spinach and season: Stir in chopped spinach and simmer for a few more minutes until the spinach wilts. Adjust seasoning if needed.

Serve: Ladle the Low FODMAP Lentil and Vegetable Soup into bowls, garnish with fresh parsley, and serve warm.

Quinoa and Veggie Stir-Fry

Ingredients:

1 cup quinoa, rinsed

2 cups low FODMAP vegetable broth or water

1 block firm tofu, drained and cubed

2 tablespoons garlic-infused oil (for low FODMAP option)

2 cups mixed low FODMAP vegetables (bell peppers, carrots, bok choy, etc.), sliced

1 tablespoon low-sodium soy sauce (for gluten-free, ensure it's low FODMAP)

1 tablespoon rice vinegar

1 tablespoon maple syrup

Sesame seeds for garnish (optional)

Instructions:

Prepare the quinoa: In a saucepan, combine the rinsed quinoa and low FODMAP vegetable broth or water. Bring to a boil, then reduce heat to low, cover, and simmer for 15-20 minutes or until the quinoa is cooked and the liquid is absorbed. Set aside.

Prepare the tofu: Heat 1 tablespoon of garlic-infused oil in a skillet over medium heat. Add the cubed tofu and cook until golden brown on all sides. Remove the tofu from the skillet and set it aside.

Stir-fry the vegetables: In the same skillet, add the remaining tablespoon of garlic-infused oil if needed. Stir-fry the mixed vegetables for 3-4 minutes until they are tender-crisp.

Combine tofu and vegetables: Return the cooked tofu to the skillet with the vegetables.

Make the sauce: In a small bowl, mix together the low-sodium soy sauce, rice vinegar, and maple syrup. Pour the sauce over the tofu and vegetables in the skillet. Toss everything together until well coated and heated through.

Serve: Serve the Stir-Fried Quinoa and Vegetables with tofu over cooked quinoa. Garnish with sesame seeds if desired.

Zucchini Noodles with Pesto

Ingredients:

4 medium zucchinis, spiralized or cut into noodles

1 cup fresh basil leaves

1/4 cup pine nuts (or walnuts for a low FODMAP option)

1/4 cup grated Parmesan cheese (optional or use a lactose-free alternative)

1/4 cup olive oil

1 tablespoon lemon juice

Salt and pepper to taste

Cherry tomatoes, halved (optional for garnish)

Instructions:

Prepare the zucchini noodles: Use a spiralizer or a vegetable peeler to create zucchini noodles. Set aside.

Make the pesto: In a food processor, combine the basil leaves, pine nuts (or walnuts), grated Parmesan (if using), olive oil, lemon juice, salt, and pepper. Blend until it forms a smooth pesto sauce.

Cook the zucchini noodles: In a large skillet, heat a little olive oil over medium heat. Add the zucchini noodles and sauté for 2-3 minutes until they are just tender. Be careful not to overcook—they should retain a slight crunch.

Combine with pesto: Once the noodles are cooked, add the prepared pesto sauce to the skillet and toss the noodles until they're evenly coated with the pesto.

Garnish and serve: Serve the Low FODMAP Zucchini Noodles with Pesto in bowls. You can add halved cherry tomatoes as a garnish if desired.

Sheet Pan Lemon Herb Chicken and Vegetables

Ingredients:

4 boneless, skinless chicken breasts

2 cups baby potatoes, halved

2 cups carrots, sliced into sticks

2 cups green beans, trimmed

2 tablespoons olive oil

Zest and juice of 1 lemon

2 tablespoons fresh parsley, chopped

1 tablespoon fresh thyme leaves

Salt and pepper to taste

Instructions:

Preheat the oven: Preheat your oven to 400°F (200°C).

Prepare the chicken and vegetables: Place the chicken breasts in the center of a large baking sheet. Arrange the baby potatoes, carrots, and green beans around the chicken.

Make the marinade: In a small bowl, mix together the olive oil, lemon zest, lemon juice, chopped parsley, fresh thyme leaves, salt, and pepper.

Coat the chicken and vegetables: Brush the chicken breasts and vegetables generously with the prepared marinade, ensuring they're evenly coated.

Bake: Place the baking sheet in the preheated oven and bake for about 25-30 minutes or until the chicken is cooked through and the vegetables are tender. The internal temperature of the chicken should reach 165°F (74°C).

Serve: Once done, remove from the oven and let it rest for a few minutes. Serve the Lemon Herb Chicken with roasted vegetables.

Baked Salmon with Herbed Quinoa

Ingredients:

4 salmon fillets

1 cup quinoa, rinsed

2 cups low FODMAP vegetable broth or water

2 tablespoons chopped fresh dill

2 tablespoons chopped fresh chives

2 tablespoons chopped fresh parsley

2 tablespoons olive oil

1 lemon, sliced

Salt and pepper to taste

Instructions:

Preheat the oven: Preheat your oven to 375°F (190°C).

Prepare the quinoa: In a saucepan, combine the quinoa and low FODMAP vegetable broth or water. Bring to a boil, then reduce heat to low, cover, and simmer for 15-20 minutes or until the liquid is absorbed and the quinoa is cooked. Fluff it with a fork and set aside.

Prepare the salmon: Place the salmon fillets on a baking sheet lined with parchment paper. Drizzle olive oil over the salmon and season with chopped dill, chives, parsley, salt, and pepper. Place lemon slices on top of each fillet.

Bake the salmon: Place the baking sheet in the preheated oven and bake for about 12-15 minutes or until the salmon is cooked through and flakes easily with a fork.

Serve: Serve the baked salmon alongside the herbed quinoa.

Maple Cinnamon Roasted Almonds

Ingredients:

2 cups whole almonds

2 tablespoons maple syrup (use pure maple syrup for low FODMAP)

1 teaspoon ground cinnamon

1/4 teaspoon salt

Instructions:

Preheat the oven: Preheat your oven to 300°F (150°C). Line a baking sheet with parchment paper.

Prepare the almonds: In a mixing bowl, combine the almonds, maple syrup, ground cinnamon, and salt. Toss until the almonds are evenly coated.

Roast the almonds: Spread the almonds in a single layer on the prepared baking sheet. Roast in the preheated oven for about 20-25 minutes, stirring occasionally to prevent burning. Keep an eye on them in the last few minutes as they can quickly go from toasted to burnt.

Cool and serve: Once the almonds are fragrant and golden brown, remove them from the oven and allow them to cool completely. The maple cinnamon roasted almonds can be stored in an airtight container once cooled.

Berry Chia Seed Pudding

Ingredients:

1 cup unsweetened almond milk (or lactose-free milk)

1/4 cup chia seeds

1 tablespoon maple syrup (use pure maple syrup for low FODMAP)

1/2 teaspoon vanilla extract

1 cup mixed low FODMAP berries (strawberries, blueberries, raspberries)

Instructions:

Prepare the chia pudding: In a bowl or jar, combine the almond milk, chia seeds, maple syrup, and vanilla extract. Stir well to combine. Cover the bowl or jar and refrigerate for at least

4 hours or overnight, allowing the chia seeds to absorb the liquid and form a pudding-like consistency.

Prepare the berries: Wash and slice the mixed berries.

Assemble the pudding: Once the chia seed mixture has thickened into a pudding-like consistency, spoon it into serving bowls or glasses. Top each serving with the mixed berries.

Serve: Serve the Low FODMAP Berry Chia Seed Pudding chilled.

Banana-Oat Cookies

Ingredients:

2 ripe bananas

1 cup rolled oats (ensure they're certified gluten-free if needed)

2 tablespoons unsweetened shredded coconut

2 tablespoons dark chocolate chips (check for no high FODMAP ingredients)

1 tablespoon maple syrup (use pure maple syrup for low FODMAP)

1/2 teaspoon vanilla extract

Pinch of cinnamon (optional)

Instructions:

Preheat the oven: Preheat your oven to 350°F (175°C). Line a baking sheet with parchment paper.

Mash the bananas: In a mixing bowl, mash the ripe bananas with a fork until smooth.

Add the remaining ingredients: Add rolled oats, shredded coconut, dark chocolate chips, maple syrup, vanilla extract, and a pinch of cinnamon (if using) to the mashed bananas. Stir well to combine all the ingredients.

Form cookies: Take spoonfuls of the mixture and place them onto the prepared baking sheet, shaping them into cookie shapes with the back of the spoon.

Bake the cookies: Place the baking sheet in the preheated oven and bake for 12-15 minutes or until the cookies are golden and firm.

Cool and serve: Once done, remove the cookies from the oven and let them cool on a wire rack.

Enjoy these delicious low FODMAP Banana-Oat Cookies as a guilt-free dessert or snack!

Chocolate Avocado Mousse

Ingredients:

2 ripe avocados

1/4 cup unsweetened cocoa powder

1/4 cup maple syrup (use pure maple syrup for low FODMAP)

1 teaspoon vanilla extract

Pinch of salt

Optional toppings: Fresh berries, shredded coconut, or chopped nuts (check for low FODMAP options)

Instructions:

Prepare the avocados: Cut the avocados in half, remove the pits, and scoop the flesh into a food processor or blender.

Blend ingredients: Add cocoa powder, maple syrup, vanilla extract, and a pinch of salt to the avocado in the food processor or blender. Blend until smooth and creamy, scraping down the sides as needed to ensure everything is well combined.

Chill the mousse: Transfer the chocolate avocado mixture to a bowl or individual serving cups. Cover and refrigerate for at least 30 minutes to allow the mousse to chill and set.

Serve: Once chilled, serve the Low FODMAP Chocolate Avocado Mousse topped with fresh berries, shredded coconut, or chopped nuts for added texture and flavor.

Peanut Butter Banana Ice Cream

Ingredients:

4 ripe bananas, peeled, sliced, and frozen

2 tablespoons peanut butter (ensure it's made with just peanuts and salt for low FODMAP)

1-2 tablespoons maple syrup (use pure maple syrup for low FODMAP, adjust sweetness to taste)

1 teaspoon vanilla extract

Instructions:

Freeze the bananas: Slice the ripe bananas into coins and place them in a freezer-safe container.

Freeze the banana slices for at least 4 hours or until frozen solid.

Blend ingredients: Once the bananas are frozen, place them in a food processor or blender. Add the peanut butter, maple syrup (start with 1 tablespoon), and vanilla extract.

Blend until creamy: Blend the ingredients until they form a smooth and creamy texture, stopping occasionally to scrape down the sides of the processor or blender. Taste and add more maple syrup if additional sweetness is desired.

Serve immediately: Scoop the Low FODMAP Peanut Butter Banana Ice Cream into bowls and enjoy immediately as soft-serve ice cream or transfer it to a container and freeze for a firmer texture.

Lemon Coconut Energy Balls

Ingredients:

1 cup unsweetened shredded coconut

1/2 cup almond flour

Zest of 1 lemon

Juice of 1/2 lemon

2 tablespoons maple syrup (use pure maple syrup for low FODMAP)

1 tablespoon melted coconut oil

Pinch of salt

Extra shredded coconut for rolling (optional)

Instructions:

Combine ingredients: In a mixing bowl, combine the unsweetened shredded coconut, almond flour, lemon zest, lemon juice, maple syrup, melted coconut oil, and a pinch of salt.

Mix well until the ingredients are evenly incorporated.

Form into balls: Using your hands, take small portions of the mixture and roll them into balls. If the mixture is too crumbly to form into balls, add a little more melted coconut oil to help bind it together.

Roll in shredded coconut (optional): If desired, roll the formed balls in additional shredded coconut for an extra coating.

Chill and serve: Place the Lemon Coconut Energy Balls on a plate or tray and refrigerate them for at least 30 minutes to set.

Raspberry Chia Pudding

Ingredients:

1 cup unsweetened almond milk (or lactose-free milk)

1/4 cup chia seeds

1 tablespoon maple syrup (use pure maple syrup for low FODMAP)

1/2 teaspoon vanilla extract

1/2 cup fresh raspberries (or any other low FODMAP berries)

Instructions:

Prepare the chia pudding: In a bowl or jar, mix together the almond milk, chia seeds, maple syrup, and vanilla extract. Stir well until all ingredients are combined. Cover the bowl or jar and refrigerate for at least 2 hours or overnight, allowing the chia seeds to absorb the liquid and thicken into a pudding-like consistency.

Blend the raspberries: In a blender or food processor, puree the fresh raspberries until smooth. If desired, strain the puree through a fine mesh sieve to remove seeds.

Assemble the pudding: Once the chia seed mixture has thickened into a pudding-like consistency, spoon it into serving glasses or bowls. Top the chia pudding with the raspberry puree.

Serve: Serve the Low FODMAP Raspberry Chia Pudding chilled.

Cinnamon Baked Apples

Ingredients:

4 medium-sized firm apples (such as Gala or Fuji)

2 tablespoons maple syrup (use pure maple syrup for low FODMAP)

1 tablespoon melted coconut oil or butter (for lactose-free option)

1 teaspoon ground cinnamon

1/4 teaspoon ground nutmeg (optional)

Chopped nuts (almonds, walnuts) for topping (optional)

Instructions:

Preheat the oven: Preheat your oven to 375°F (190°C).

Prepare the apples: Wash the apples thoroughly and remove the cores, creating a hollow space in the center. You can use an apple corer or a knife to carefully remove the core without cutting through the bottom of the apples.

Mix the filling: In a small bowl, mix together the maple syrup, melted coconut oil or butter, ground cinnamon, and ground nutmeg (if using).

Fill the apples: Place the cored apples on a baking dish or tray. Spoon the cinnamon mixture into each apple, distributing it evenly among them.

Bake the apples: Bake the apples in the preheated oven for about 25-30 minutes or until they are tender and lightly browned.

Serve: Once baked, remove the apples from the oven and let them cool slightly. You can optionally sprinkle chopped nuts on top for added texture.

Chocolate-Dipped Strawberries

Ingredients:

1 pint fresh strawberries, rinsed and dried

4 ounces dark chocolate (check for no high FODMAP ingredients), chopped

1 tablespoon coconut oil

Optional toppings: Crushed nuts (such as almonds or pecans), shredded coconut (unsweetened), or sea salt flakes

Instructions:

Prepare the strawberries: Line a baking sheet or tray with parchment paper. Ensure the strawberries are thoroughly dried after rinsing to allow the chocolate to stick better.

Melt the chocolate: In a microwave-safe bowl or using a double boiler, melt the dark chocolate and coconut oil together in short intervals, stirring frequently until smooth and fully melted.

Dip the strawberries: Holding each strawberry by the stem, dip it into the melted chocolate, swirling to coat about two-thirds of the berry. Allow any excess chocolate to drip off.

Add toppings (optional): If desired, immediately sprinkle the dipped strawberries with crushed nuts, shredded coconut, or a pinch of sea salt flakes before the chocolate sets.

Set and chill: Place the chocolate-dipped strawberries onto the prepared baking sheet. Refrigerate them for about 15-20 minutes or until the chocolate is set.

Serve: Once the chocolate is firm, arrange the Low FODMAP Chocolate-Dipped Strawberries on a plate and serve as a delightful dessert.

Coconut Rice Pudding

Ingredients:

1 cup Arborio rice (or sushi rice)

2 cups unsweetened coconut milk

2 cups water

1/4 cup maple syrup (use pure maple syrup for low FODMAP)

1 teaspoon vanilla extract

1/2 cup unsweetened shredded coconut

Ground cinnamon for garnish (optional)

Instructions:

Rinse and cook the rice: Rinse the Arborio rice under cold water until the water runs clear. In a saucepan, combine the rinsed rice, coconut milk, water, maple syrup, and vanilla extract. Bring the mixture to a boil over medium heat, then reduce heat to low, cover, and simmer for about 30-35 minutes, stirring occasionally, until the rice is tender and the liquid is absorbed.

Add shredded coconut: Stir in the unsweetened shredded coconut into the cooked rice pudding and let it simmer for an additional 5-7 minutes to incorporate the flavors.

Cool and serve: Remove the rice pudding from heat and let it cool for a few minutes. Serve the Low FODMAP Coconut Rice Pudding warm or chilled in individual bowls. Optionally, sprinkle ground cinnamon on top for garnish.

Almond Butter Cookies

Ingredients:

1 cup almond flour

1/4 cup smooth almond butter (check for no added high FODMAP ingredients)

2 tablespoons maple syrup (use pure maple syrup for low FODMAP)

1 teaspoon vanilla extract

Pinch of salt

Sliced almonds for garnish (optional)

Instructions:

Preheat the oven: Preheat your oven to 350°F (175°C). Line a baking sheet with parchment paper.

Mix ingredients: In a mixing bowl, combine the almond flour, smooth almond butter, maple syrup, vanilla extract, and a pinch of salt. Mix until a dough forms.

Shape the cookies: Take tablespoon-sized portions of the dough and roll them into balls. Place them on the prepared baking sheet and flatten them slightly with the palm of your hand. Optionally, press a few sliced almonds onto the top of each cookie for decoration.

Bake: Place the baking sheet in the preheated oven and bake for 10-12 minutes or until the edges of the cookies are golden brown.

Cool and serve: Once done, remove the cookies from the oven and let them cool on the baking sheet for a few minutes before transferring them to a wire rack to cool completely.

Pineapple Coconut Ice Pops

Ingredients:

1 cup fresh pineapple chunks (ensure the portion size aligns with low FODMAP recommendations)

1 cup unsweetened coconut milk

2 tablespoons maple syrup (use pure maple syrup for low FODMAP)

1 teaspoon vanilla extract

Instructions:

Blend the ingredients: In a blender, combine the fresh pineapple chunks, unsweetened coconut milk, maple syrup, and vanilla extract. Blend until smooth.

Pour into molds: Pour the pineapple-coconut mixture into ice pop molds, leaving a little space at the top for expansion. If your molds have sticks, insert them into the mixture.

Freeze: Place the filled ice pop molds in the freezer for at least 4-6 hours or until completely frozen.

Serve: Once frozen, remove the molds from the freezer. To release the ice pops, run the molds briefly under warm water or follow the instructions for your specific mold type.

Mango Sorbet

Ingredients:

2 ripe mangoes, peeled and diced

1-2 tablespoons maple syrup (use pure maple syrup for low FODMAP), optional depending on sweetness of mangoes

1-2 tablespoons freshly squeezed lime juice

1/4 cup water, if needed for blending

Instructions:

Prepare the mangoes: Peel the ripe mangoes and dice the flesh, discarding the pit.

Blend the ingredients: In a blender or food processor, combine the diced mangoes, maple syrup (if using), and freshly squeezed lime juice. Blend until smooth. If the mixture is too thick to blend, add a little water, a tablespoon at a time, until it blends smoothly.

Taste and adjust: Taste the mixture and adjust the sweetness or tanginess by adding more maple syrup or lime juice, according to your preference.

Freeze the sorbet: Pour the blended mango mixture into a shallow, freezer-safe dish. Cover the dish and place it in the freezer for about 4-6 hours, stirring every hour or so with a fork to break up any ice crystals that form. This helps create a smoother sorbet texture.

Serve: Once the sorbet has reached the desired consistency, scoop it into bowls or serving dishes. Garnish with a slice of lime or a few pieces of fresh mango if desired.

Raspberry Coconut Chia Pudding Parfait

Ingredients:

1 cup unsweetened coconut milk

1/4 cup chia seeds

1 tablespoon maple syrup (use pure maple syrup for low FODMAP)

1/2 teaspoon vanilla extract

1 cup fresh raspberries

Unsweetened shredded coconut for garnish (optional)

Instructions:

Prepare the chia pudding: In a mixing bowl or jar, combine the unsweetened coconut milk, chia seeds, maple syrup, and vanilla extract. Stir well to mix all ingredients thoroughly. Cover the bowl or jar and refrigerate for at least 2-3 hours or overnight, allowing the chia seeds to absorb the liquid and form a pudding-like consistency.

Blend the raspberries: In a blender or food processor, puree the fresh raspberries until smooth. Optionally, strain the puree through a fine mesh sieve to remove seeds if desired.

Assemble the parfait: Once the chia pudding has set, take serving glasses or jars. Spoon a layer of the chia pudding into each glass, followed by a layer of the raspberry puree. Repeat the layers until the glasses are filled, ending with a layer of raspberry puree on top.

Garnish and serve: Optionally, sprinkle unsweetened shredded coconut on top for garnish. Serve the Low FODMAP Raspberry Coconut Chia Pudding Parfait immediately or refrigerate until ready to serve.

Banana Almond Bites

Ingredients:

2 ripe bananas

1/2 cup almond flour

2 tablespoons pure maple syrup

1 teaspoon vanilla extract

Pinch of cinnamon (optional)

Sliced almonds for garnish (optional)

Instructions:

Preheat the oven: Preheat your oven to 350°F (175°C). Line a baking sheet with parchment paper.

Prepare the bananas: Peel the ripe bananas and mash them in a mixing bowl until smooth.

Mix the ingredients: To the mashed bananas, add almond flour, maple syrup, vanilla extract, and a pinch of cinnamon (if using). Stir until well combined.

Form the bites: Using a spoon or cookie scoop, form small balls or bite-sized portions from the mixture and place them on the prepared baking sheet.

Garnish (optional): Optionally, press a sliced almond onto the top of each bite for added texture and decoration.

Bake: Place the baking sheet in the preheated oven and bake for 12-15 minutes or until the bites are set and lightly golden.

Cool and serve: Once done, remove the banana almond bites from the oven and let them cool on a wire rack before serving.

Berry and Mint Salad

Ingredients:

2 cups mixed low FODMAP berries (such as strawberries, blueberries, raspberries)

1 tablespoon fresh mint leaves, thinly sliced

1 tablespoon pure maple syrup (adjust quantity based on sweetness of berries)

Zest and juice of 1 lime

Instructions:

Prepare the berries: Rinse and pat dry the mixed berries. If using strawberries, remove the stems and slice them into halves or quarters, depending on their size.

Mix the salad: In a mixing bowl, combine the mixed berries, thinly sliced fresh mint leaves, maple syrup, lime zest, and lime juice. Gently toss the ingredients together until the berries are coated evenly.

Chill and serve: Cover the bowl and refrigerate the berry and mint salad for at least 30 minutes to allow the flavors to meld.

Serve: After chilling, serve the Low FODMAP Berry and Mint Salad in individual bowls or glasses as a refreshing and naturally sweet dessert.

SOUP LOW-FODMAP DIET RECIPES

Carrot and Ginger Soup

Ingredients:

1 tablespoon olive oil

1 pound (about 450g) carrots, peeled and chopped

1 medium potato, peeled and diced

1-inch piece fresh ginger, peeled and grated

4 cups low FODMAP vegetable broth

Salt and pepper to taste

Fresh chives (green parts only) for garnish (optional)

Instructions:

Saute the vegetables: In a large pot, heat the olive oil over medium heat. Add the chopped carrots, diced potato, and grated ginger. Saute for about 5 minutes, stirring occasionally.

Add broth and simmer: Pour in the low FODMAP vegetable broth, ensuring it covers the vegetables. Bring the mixture to a boil, then reduce the heat to low. Cover the pot and simmer for 20-25 minutes or until the carrots and potato are tender.

Blend the soup: Once the vegetables are soft, remove the pot from heat and allow the soup to cool slightly. Use an immersion blender or transfer the soup in batches to a blender, and blend until smooth and creamy.

Season and serve: Return the blended soup to the pot and reheat if necessary. Season with salt and pepper to taste. If desired, garnish each serving with chopped fresh chives.

Quinoa and Vegetable Soup

Ingredients:

1 tablespoon olive oil

1 cup carrots, diced

1 cup zucchini, diced

1 cup red bell pepper, diced

1 cup cooked quinoa

4 cups low FODMAP vegetable broth

1 teaspoon dried oregano

1 teaspoon dried thyme

Salt and pepper to taste

Fresh parsley for garnish (optional)

Instructions:

Saute the vegetables: In a large pot, heat olive oil over medium heat. Add diced carrots, zucchini, and red bell pepper. Saute for about 5-7 minutes until the vegetables start to soften.

Add quinoa and broth: Stir in the cooked quinoa, low FODMAP vegetable broth, dried oregano, and dried thyme. Bring the mixture to a boil, then reduce the heat to a simmer.

Simmer and season: Let the soup simmer for 15-20 minutes until the vegetables are tender. Season with salt and pepper to taste.

Serve: Ladle the Low FODMAP Quinoa and Vegetable Soup into bowls. Garnish with fresh parsley if desired and serve warm.

Lemon Sorbet

Ingredients:

1 cup water

1/2 cup pure maple syrup (for a sweeter sorbet, adjust the quantity as desired)

Zest of 2 lemons

1 cup freshly squeezed lemon juice (from about 4-6 lemons)

Instructions:

Prepare the syrup: In a saucepan, combine water and maple syrup. Bring the mixture to a gentle boil, stirring occasionally. Once boiling, remove it from heat and let it cool to room temperature.

Prepare the lemon mixture: In a bowl, combine the lemon zest and freshly squeezed lemon juice.

Combine the mixtures: Once the syrup has cooled, mix it with the lemon juice and zest mixture. Stir well to combine.

Chill and churn: Pour the mixture into an ice cream maker and churn according to the manufacturer's instructions until it reaches a sorbet-like consistency.

Freeze: Transfer the churned sorbet into a freezer-safe container. Cover it and freeze for at least 4-6 hours or until it's firm enough to scoop.

Serve: Scoop the Low FODMAP Lemon Sorbet into serving bowls or cones. Enjoy this refreshing and tangy treat!

Tomato Basil Soup

Ingredients:

2 tablespoons olive oil

1 cup carrots, diced

1 cup celery, diced

2 cups canned crushed tomatoes (check for no high FODMAP ingredients)

4 cups low FODMAP vegetable broth

1 teaspoon dried basil

Salt and pepper to taste

Fresh basil leaves for garnish (optional)

Instructions:

Saute vegetables: In a large pot, heat olive oil over medium heat. Add diced carrots and celery. Saute for about 5-7 minutes until the vegetables soften.

Add tomatoes and broth: Pour in the canned crushed tomatoes and low FODMAP vegetable broth. Stir well to combine.

Season and simmer: Add the dried basil, salt, and pepper. Bring the mixture to a simmer. Reduce the heat and let it simmer uncovered for 15-20 minutes, allowing the flavors to meld.

Blend (optional): For a smoother texture, use an immersion blender or transfer the soup in batches to a blender and blend until smooth.

Serve: Ladle the Low FODMAP Tomato Basil Soup into bowls. Garnish with fresh basil leaves if desired and serve warm.

Butternut Squash Soup

Ingredients:

1 medium butternut squash, peeled, seeded, and diced (about 4 cups)

1 tablespoon olive oil

1 cup carrots, diced

1 cup potatoes, peeled and diced

4 cups low FODMAP vegetable broth

1 teaspoon ground cumin

1/2 teaspoon ground cinnamon

Salt and pepper to taste

Fresh chives (green parts only) for garnish (optional)

Instructions:

Roast the squash: Preheat your oven to 400°F (200°C). Place the diced butternut squash on a baking sheet, drizzle with olive oil, and season lightly with salt. Roast for about 25-30 minutes or until the squash is tender and slightly caramelized. Remove from the oven and set aside.

Saute vegetables: In a large pot, heat olive oil over medium heat. Add diced carrots and potatoes. Saute for about 5-7 minutes until they begin to soften.

Add roasted squash and broth: Add the roasted butternut squash to the pot along with the low FODMAP vegetable broth. Stir well.

Season and simmer: Stir in the ground cumin, ground cinnamon, salt, and pepper. Bring the mixture to a boil, then reduce the heat and let it simmer for 15-20 minutes, allowing the flavors to meld.

Blend (optional): Use an immersion blender or transfer the soup in batches to a blender and blend until smooth.

Serve: Ladle the Low FODMAP Butternut Squash Soup into bowls. Garnish with fresh chives if desired and serve warm.

Spinach and Potato Soup

Ingredients:

1 tablespoon olive oil

2 cups potatoes, peeled and diced

1 cup carrots, diced

1 cup spinach, chopped

4 cups low FODMAP vegetable broth

1 teaspoon dried thyme

Salt and pepper to taste

Fresh parsley for garnish (optional)

Instructions:

Saute vegetables: In a large pot, heat olive oil over medium heat. Add diced potatoes and carrots. Saute for about 5-7 minutes until they start to soften.

Add broth and simmer: Pour in the low FODMAP vegetable broth and chopped spinach. Stir well. Add dried thyme, salt, and pepper. Bring the mixture to a boil, then reduce the heat and let it simmer for 15-20 minutes or until the vegetables are tender.

Blend (optional): For a smoother consistency, use an immersion blender or transfer a portion of the soup to a blender and blend until desired smoothness. Return it to the pot and mix well.

Serve: Ladle the Low FODMAP Spinach and Potato Soup into bowls. Garnish with fresh parsley if desired and serve warm.

Lentil and Vegetable Soup

Ingredients:

1 tablespoon olive oil

1 cup carrots, diced

1 cup zucchini, diced

1 cup bell peppers (red or yellow), diced

1 cup diced tomatoes (canned or fresh)

1 cup dry lentils, rinsed and drained

6 cups low FODMAP vegetable broth

1 teaspoon dried thyme

1 teaspoon ground cumin

Salt and pepper to taste

Fresh parsley for garnish (optional)

Instructions:

Saute vegetables: In a large pot, heat olive oil over medium heat. Add diced carrots, zucchini, and bell peppers. Saute for about 5 minutes until they start to soften.

Add lentils and broth: Add diced tomatoes, rinsed lentils, low FODMAP vegetable broth, dried thyme, and ground cumin to the pot. Stir well.

Simmer: Bring the mixture to a boil, then reduce the heat to a simmer. Cover and let it cook for about 25-30 minutes or until the lentils and vegetables are tender.

Season: Season the soup with salt and pepper to taste.

Serve: Ladle the Low FODMAP Lentil and Vegetable Soup into bowls. Garnish with fresh parsley if desired and serve hot.

Broccoli and Potato Soup

Ingredients:

1 tablespoon olive oil

2 cups broccoli florets

2 cups potatoes, peeled and diced

1 cup carrots, diced

4 cups low FODMAP vegetable broth

1 teaspoon dried thyme

Salt and pepper to taste

Fresh chives (green parts only) for garnish (optional)

Instructions:

Saute vegetables: In a large pot, heat olive oil over medium heat. Add diced potatoes and carrots. Saute for about 5 minutes until they start to soften.

Add broth and broccoli: Pour in the low FODMAP vegetable broth. Add broccoli florets and dried thyme. Stir well.

Simmer: Bring the mixture to a boil, then reduce the heat to a simmer. Cover and let it cook for about 15-20 minutes or until the vegetables are tender.

Blend (optional): For a creamier texture, use an immersion blender or transfer a portion of the soup to a blender and blend until desired consistency. Return it to the pot and mix well.

Season: Season the soup with salt and pepper to taste.

Serve: Ladle the Low FODMAP Broccoli and Potato Soup into bowls. Garnish with fresh chives if desired and serve warm.

Spiced Pumpkin Soup

Ingredients:

1 tablespoon olive oil

1 cup canned pumpkin puree (ensure no high FODMAP ingredients)

2 cups carrots, peeled and chopped

1 cup parsnips, peeled and chopped

4 cups low FODMAP vegetable broth

1 teaspoon ground cumin

1/2 teaspoon ground ginger

1/4 teaspoon ground nutmeg

Salt and pepper to taste

Fresh parsley for garnish (optional)

Instructions:

Saute vegetables: In a large pot, heat olive oil over medium heat. Add chopped carrots and parsnips. Saute for about 5-7 minutes until they start to soften.

Add pumpkin and broth: Stir in the canned pumpkin puree, low FODMAP vegetable broth, ground cumin, ground ginger, and ground nutmeg. Mix well.

Simmer: Bring the mixture to a boil, then reduce the heat to a simmer. Cover and let it cook for about 20-25 minutes or until the vegetables are tender.

Blend (optional): For a smoother texture, use an immersion blender or transfer a portion of the soup to a blender and blend until desired consistency. Return it to the pot and mix well.

Season: Season the soup with salt and pepper to taste.

Serve: Ladle the Low FODMAP Spiced Pumpkin Soup into bowls. Garnish with fresh parsley if desired and serve warm.

Roasted Red Pepper Soup

Ingredients:

4 red bell peppers

1 tablespoon olive oil

1 cup carrots, diced

1 cup potatoes, diced

4 cups low FODMAP vegetable broth

1 teaspoon dried basil

1/2 teaspoon smoked paprika

Salt and pepper to taste

Fresh basil leaves for garnish (optional)

Instructions:

Roast the bell peppers: Preheat the oven to 400°F (200°C). Place the whole red bell peppers on a baking sheet and roast them in the oven for about 25-30 minutes, turning occasionally, until the skin is charred and blistered. Remove from the oven and let them cool. Once cooled, peel off the skin, remove seeds, and chop the roasted peppers.

Saute vegetables: In a large pot, heat olive oil over medium heat. Add diced carrots and potatoes. Saute for about 5 minutes until they start to soften.

Add broth and roasted peppers: Pour in the low FODMAP vegetable broth and add the chopped roasted red peppers. Stir well.

Season and simmer: Add dried basil, smoked paprika, salt, and pepper. Bring the mixture to a boil, then reduce the heat to a simmer. Cover and let it cook for about 15-20 minutes or until the vegetables are tender.

Blend (optional): For a smoother texture, use an immersion blender or transfer a portion of the soup to a blender and blend until desired consistency. Return it to the pot and mix well.

Serve: Ladle the Low FODMAP Roasted Red Pepper Soup into bowls. Garnish with fresh basil leaves if desired and serve warm.

Lemon Chicken Soup

Ingredients:

1 tablespoon olive oil

2 boneless, skinless chicken breasts, diced

1 cup carrots, diced

1 cup celery, diced

6 cups low FODMAP chicken broth

Zest and juice of 1 lemon

1 teaspoon dried thyme

Salt and pepper to taste

Fresh parsley for garnish (optional)

Instructions:

Saute chicken and vegetables: In a large pot, heat olive oil over medium heat. Add diced chicken breasts and cook until lightly browned. Add diced carrots and celery. Saute for about 5 minutes until the vegetables begin to soften.

Add broth and seasonings: Pour in the low FODMAP chicken broth. Add the lemon zest, lemon juice, dried thyme, salt, and pepper. Stir well.

Simmer: Bring the mixture to a boil, then reduce the heat to a simmer. Cover and let it cook for about 15-20 minutes or until the chicken is cooked through and the vegetables are tender.

Serve: Ladle the Low FODMAP Lemon Chicken Soup into bowls. Garnish with fresh parsley if desired and serve hot.

Thai-Inspired Shrimp Soup

Ingredients:

1 tablespoon sesame oil

1-inch piece of fresh ginger, peeled and minced

2 cups bok choy, chopped

1 cup carrots, sliced

1 cup red bell pepper, sliced

1 can (13.5 oz) unsweetened coconut milk

4 cups low FODMAP seafood or vegetable broth

1 tablespoon low FODMAP red curry paste

1 tablespoon fish sauce (check for no high FODMAP ingredients)

1 pound shrimp, peeled and deveined

Juice of 1 lime

Fresh cilantro for garnish (optional)

Instructions:

Saute aromatics and vegetables: In a large pot, heat sesame oil over medium heat. Add minced ginger and sauté for a minute. Add bok choy, carrots, and red bell pepper. Cook for about 5 minutes until vegetables begin to soften.

Add coconut milk and broth: Pour in the unsweetened coconut milk and low FODMAP seafood or vegetable broth. Stir well.

Add curry paste and fish sauce: Add the red curry paste and fish sauce to the pot, stirring until well combined.

Cook shrimp: Add the peeled and deveined shrimp to the soup. Cook for about 3-5 minutes or until the shrimp turn pink and opaque.

Finish with lime juice: Squeeze the juice of 1 lime into the soup and stir.

Serve: Ladle the Low FODMAP Thai-Inspired Shrimp Soup into bowls. Garnish with fresh cilantro if desired and serve hot.

Zucchini and Basil Soup

Ingredients:

1 tablespoon olive oil

4 cups zucchini, diced

1 cup leek (green parts only), chopped

2 cups low FODMAP vegetable broth

1 cup spinach leaves

1/4 cup fresh basil leaves

Salt and pepper to taste

Lemon zest for garnish (optional)

Instructions:

Saute vegetables: In a large pot, heat olive oil over medium heat. Add diced zucchini and chopped leek (green parts only). Saute for about 5-7 minutes until they begin to soften.

Add broth and simmer: Pour in the low FODMAP vegetable broth. Bring the mixture to a boil, then reduce the heat to a simmer. Let it cook for about 10-12 minutes or until the zucchini is tender.

Add spinach and basil: Stir in the spinach leaves and fresh basil leaves. Cook for an additional 2-3 minutes until the spinach wilts.

Blend the soup: Remove the pot from heat. Using an immersion blender or transferring in batches to a blender, blend the soup until smooth.

Season: Return the blended soup to the pot. Season with salt and pepper to taste.

Serve: Ladle the Low FODMAP Zucchini and Basil Soup into bowls. Optionally, garnish with a sprinkle of lemon zest for added flavor and serve warm.

Lentil Soup

Ingredients:

1 tablespoon olive oil

1 cup carrots, diced

1 cup celery, diced

1 cup potatoes, diced

1 cup canned lentils, drained and rinsed

4 cups low FODMAP vegetable broth

1 teaspoon dried thyme

1 bay leaf

Salt and pepper to taste

Fresh parsley for garnish (optional)

Instructions:

Saute vegetables: In a large pot, heat olive oil over medium heat. Add diced carrots, celery, and potatoes. Saute for about 5 minutes until they start to soften.

Add lentils and broth: Add the canned lentils (previously drained and rinsed) to the pot. Pour in the low FODMAP vegetable broth. Stir well.

Season and simmer: Add dried thyme, a bay leaf, salt, and pepper. Bring the mixture to a boil, then reduce the heat to a simmer. Cover and let it cook for about 20-25 minutes or until the vegetables are tender.

Serve: Remove the bay leaf before serving. Ladle the Low FODMAP Lentil Soup into bowls. Garnish with fresh parsley if desired and serve hot.

Egg Drop Soup

Ingredients:

4 cups low FODMAP chicken broth

2 eggs

2 tablespoons cornstarch (or tapioca starch)

2 tablespoons water

1 teaspoon sesame oil

2 green onions (green parts only), finely chopped

Salt and pepper to taste

Instructions:

Prepare thickening mixture: In a small bowl, mix cornstarch (or tapioca starch) with water until fully dissolved.

Heat broth: In a pot, bring low FODMAP chicken broth to a gentle simmer over medium heat.

Whisk eggs: In a separate bowl, beat the eggs until well mixed.

Add thickening mixture: Slowly pour the cornstarch mixture into the simmering broth while stirring constantly. This will thicken the soup slightly.

Add eggs: While stirring the broth in a circular motion, slowly pour in the beaten eggs. This will create the characteristic egg ribbons in the soup. Cook for about 1 minute.

Season and finish: Add sesame oil, chopped green onions (green parts only), salt, and pepper. Adjust seasoning according to taste.

Serve: Ladle the Low FODMAP Egg Drop Soup into bowls and serve hot.

Chicken and Rice Soup

Ingredients:

1 tablespoon olive oil

2 boneless, skinless chicken breasts, diced

1 cup carrots, diced

1 cup celery, diced

1 cup cooked rice (use low FODMAP variety)

6 cups low FODMAP chicken broth

1 teaspoon dried thyme

Salt and pepper to taste

Fresh parsley for garnish (optional)

Instructions:

Saute chicken and vegetables: In a large pot, heat olive oil over medium heat. Add diced chicken breasts and cook until lightly browned. Add diced carrots and celery. Saute for about 5 minutes until they start to soften.

Add broth and rice: Pour in the low FODMAP chicken broth. Add the cooked rice and dried thyme. Stir well.

Simmer: Bring the mixture to a boil, then reduce the heat to a simmer. Let it cook for about 15-20 minutes or until the vegetables are tender.

Season: Season the soup with salt and pepper to taste.

Serve: Ladle the Low FODMAP Chicken and Rice Soup into bowls. Optionally, garnish with fresh parsley and serve hot.